Generation Rx

Generation Rx

HOW PRESCRIPTION DRUGS
ARE ALTERING AMERICAN LIVES,
MINDS, AND BODIES

Greg Critser

A MARINER BOOK
HOUGHTON MIFFLIN COMPANY
BOSTON • NEW YORK

FOR MY MOTHER, BETTY CRITSER

First Mariner Books edition 2006
Copyright © 2005 by Greg Critser

For information about permission to reproduce selections
from this book, write to Permissions, Houghton Mifflin Company,
215 Park Avenue South, New York, New York 10003.

Visit our Web site: www.houghtonmifflinbooks.com.

Library of Congress Cataloging-in-Publication Data
Critser, Greg.
Generation Rx : how prescription drugs are altering
American lives, minds, and bodies / Greg Critser.
p. ; cm.
Includes index.
ISBN-13: 978-0-618-39313-8   ISBN-10: 0-618-39313-7
1. Drug utilization—United States. 2. Pharmaceutical industry—United
States. 3. Drugs—Social aspects—United States. [DNLM: 1. Drug Industry
—economics—United States—Popular Works. 2. Health Behavior—
United States—Popular Works. 3. Health Policy—United States—Popular
Works. 4. Population Groups—psychology—United States—Popular
Works. QV 736 C934g 2005] I. Title.
RM263.C75 2005   338.4'76151—dc22   2005009113
ISBN-13: 978-0-618-77356-5 (pbk.)
ISBN-10: 0-618-77356-8 (pbk.)

Printed in the United States of America

Book design by Robert Overholtzer

QUM 10 9 8 7 6 5 4 3 2 1

Contents

Acknowledgments

Generation Rx is the product of a decade-long interest in the marketing of prescription drugs, and it has benefited greatly from the advice, wisdom, generosity, and courage of a number of individuals. Colin Harrison, my editor at *Harper's,* was the first to pay me to write about the subject; our wide-ranging discussions planted the invaluable seeds of the book more than thirteen years ago. Dan Ferrara, my editor at *Worth,* pushed my interest along by publishing a lengthy (and, for a business magazine, no-holds-barred) essay about my interviews with drug-company executives. That article also benefited from Dean Robinson's deft editing. At the *Los Angeles Times,* Sue Horton was a consistent, unyielding source of good editorial judgment, and she also bought me lunch. Thanks. At *USA Today,* Glenn Nishimura published several of my early op-ed pieces on the subject, and for that I am grateful too.

Generation Rx has also prospered from the insights of a number of unofficial advisers, mentors, and intellectual provocateurs. William Vodra, an attorney at Arnold and Porter, was an acute and generous industry observer who took the time to explain why things happened the way they did in the nation's capital. Al Engelberg, who litigated the first great generic drug cases, was similarly beneficent, patient, and thoughtful. Larry Sasich, at Public Citizen, provided a number of key interviews, his fair-minded assessments further proof that on any given day his and Sidney Wolfe's work on drug safety remains *the* ethical standard and the patient's best friend. John Kamp, at the law firm of Wiley Rein, was an outstanding tutor on media law and FDA regulation. In the sphere of medicine and pharmacological science, I was fortunate as well. Here my Virgil was UCLA's Dr. Barbara Levey, the past president of the American Society of Clinical Pharmacology and Therapeutics and a leading mover in the effort to get better science into the hands of prescribing physicians.

A book like this doesn't get far without the coddling, coaxing, tending, and care of two other critical players, an agent and an editor, and here again I find myself blessed. Richard Abate, at ICM, is a great agent, sagacious and literate. Deanne Urmy, my editor at Houghton Mifflin, was an unwavering source of support, wisdom, and advice — without which the scale of the book would not have been possible. Also, she laughs at my jokes, and she knows how to ride a horse.

Any originality I brought to the subject was aided by a number of individuals, among whom were Ted C. Fishman, Daniel Fineman, Barry Sanders, Mark Salzman, Joel Kotkin, Jeremy Newman, Steve Oney, Nancy Wadsworth, Catherine Seipp, Wolfgang Neuman, Robert Lerner, and Francine Kaufman. Ditto Jessica, Connie, and John Yu. Over the long term, the book and I benefited immeasurably from the counsel of James Stillwell, Robert Holmes, Robert Spear, Ben Weidenbener, and Ed Burke. The staff of UCLA's Louise M. Darling Biomedical Library were, as always, helpful, patient, and thoughtful, as were the staff at the National Archives in College Park, Maryland. During the actual writing and production of *Generation Rx,* Fiona Cole made footnoting (almost) fun, while the crew at Yoga House kept me in the psychic saddle. And then there was the great horseman Jeff Peters, who kept me in the literal one. Heels down!

In the realm of daily book writing, family truly matters the most. *Generation Rx* was deepened by my constant interaction with my mother-in-law, Julia Mongelli, and especially my father-in-law, Rocky Mongelli, who has, through his own harrowing adventures as a patient, made me see the questions that really count. My mother, Betty Critser, to whom this book is dedicated, was unflagging in her support for my writing — something I could not get along without. My wife, Antoinette Mongelli, once again braved the endless waves of writerly self-absorption with grace and kindness, and she has given *Generation Rx* its heart.

Generation Rx

Introduction

When a great profession and the forces of capitalism interact,
drama is likely to result.

— David Blumenthal, M.D.,
Massachusetts General Hospital

NOT LONG AGO, while reading through the pages of the *New
York Times*, I came upon an article that really grabbed me, not
because it was about some new horror abroad or another political
debacle at home, but rather because it limned so cleanly the way
American lives are changing. It was a story in the paper's "House
and Home" section about the rise in popularity of "triple-wide"
medicine cabinets. As the *Times* put it, "First there were French
fries. Then there were sport utility vehicles. Now even the most
private of domestic preserves, the medicine cabinet, has been
supersized. With the sales of lotions, potions, 'nutraceuticals'
and pharmaceuticals climbing to new heights, manufacturers
are responding with medicine cabinets that are taller, wider and
deeper than ever before."

The article included photographs of the classic bathroom cabinet — the tiny stained wall-hanger that most of us grew up with
— and a slew of the new breed: the "floor-to-ceiling," the "walk-
in," the "super-deep and super-wide." There were cabinets with
built-in defoggers and others hinged with fancy rubber gaskets so
that they don't go "click" when one doesn't want them to go
click. The designers' ingenuity was stunning, the new owners'
justifications for their triple-wides quirky or peevish. ("He's

obsessed with muscle power pills!" complained one woman of her husband's quest for more medicine chest space.) Everybody wanted bigger ones, better ones.

This book is about the products taking up an increasingly huge and expensive chunk of space in that American medicine chest: prescription drugs. Unlike potions and lotions for one's skin and hair, they are not products that we "decide" we want. Prescription drugs are products that highly educated people, whom we trust with our money and our lives, tell us that *we need in order to survive or to avoid undue risk to our health.*

Over the past decade the use of these drugs, almost all for chronic diseases, has soared. The average number of prescriptions per person, annually, in 1993 was seven. The average number of prescriptions per person, annually, in 2000 was eleven. In 2004, it was twelve. The total number of annual prescriptions in the United States now stands at about 3 billion. The cost per year? About $180 billion, headed to an estimated $414 billion by 2011. Pretty soon, as the saying goes, you are talking real money.

There's another number to consider: In 2004, almost half of all Americans used at least one prescription drug on a *daily* basis; amazingly, about one in six take three or more a day. That represents a substantial rise from the early 1980s, when Americans — patients and physicians alike — seemed much more leery about using new drugs. Such is no longer the case. Today, Americans are more willing than ever to experiment, or, more precisely, to be experimented upon.

Today the expectation is that pills can and will do everything, from guarding us against our excesses of drink, food, and tobacco, to increasing our children's performance at school, to jump-starting our own productivity at work, to extending our very time on this mortal coil. Indeed pills — and by that I mean prescription drugs that require a physician's signed authorization — have become interwoven with the very notion of what constitutes health. In a strange and trusting way, we see them not as cures so much as partners — their message about why they work in, say, reducing cholesterol or lowering blood pressure being almost as important as the pill itself. It is hard not to note the irony: the generation of Americans who rebelliously experimented with drugs is now a generation upon whom drugs are experimented, with barely a squeak of protest. Call us Generation Rx.

Our trust in prescriptions persists even in the face of enormous uncertainty about many drugs' benefits and safety. Consider the continuing debate about antidepressants and children, which fills the pages of daily newspapers as well as medical journals and countless Internet sites, pro and con (but almost never in between). On one day during the summer of 2004, readers of the *New York Times* were told, on the front page, that such drugs are effective for kids; on the very next day, on the front page again, they were told that the attorney general of New York was suing the maker of one such antidepressant for fraudulently covering up safety and efficacy problems, including suicide, in children using the drugs. Other classes of drugs have also come under deep scrutiny, most notably pills for arthritis known as COX-2 inhibitors; last autumn Merck was forced to recall its huge-selling Vioxx for causing, by one count, somewhere between 56,000 and 100,000 heart attacks. Similar, albeit less publicized, uncertainties exist with a number of other widely used drugs, yet our rate of usage continues to spiral upward.

Why is that? Is it because Americans today are a more acquiescent breed than they were a generation ago? Perhaps, although you'd get an earful in the red states for uttering that heresy. Or is it because we are more stressed, with bodies that cry out for new and better ameliorating agents? That might be part of the stew as well. Or is it because we have been put between a rock and a hard place? To wit: Has managed care, with its stingy allocation of resources for face-to-face medicine, made pills the de facto primary care physician, Dr. Merck, M.D.? Certainly physicians themselves have become more willing to prescribe new drugs, not to mention the growing numbers who are quite comfortable prescribing pills for totally untested and unapproved uses. Why is that? And why do we take them? Does our trust in our physicians' prescriptions come out of desperation or from something else, like a lack of clear communication about risks and benefits — risks and benefits that get drowned out by the constant promotional bombardment from the pharmaceutical industry, a.k.a. big pharma?

I was reminded of that complicated reality not long ago, when accompanying Rocky, my seventy-five-year-old father-in-law, to a series of medical appointments at Los Angeles County–University of Southern California Medical Center, a world-class treatment and research hospital. Because of a transfusion of bad blood more than thirty years ago, Rocky has hepatitis C; the virus has caused scarring on parts of his liver. On and off, his liver "panels" — tests for excess "bad" enzymes and the like — shoot up and down. Yet he remains asymptomatic — he does not have jaundice and he is not affected in his daily life. His liver specialist once tried to kill the virus using interferon, a powerful chemical that not only failed at the mission, but rendered my father-in-law deeply depressed, twenty-five pounds overweight, nearly narcoleptic. He went off the drug and returned to normal. But that wasn't the end of it. A few months later, his specialist asked him to come in. This doctor was getting bombed with pharmaceutical company–funded requests for subjects in a clinical trial for hep C, this one involving a combination of interferon and another drug. He suggested that Rocky check it out.

At USC, we learned from one of the head investigators that the prospect of the combination working was slim. Still, it was "state of the art." All through the screening process, I kept asking Rocky, Did he understand what the USC researchers were saying? This was an experiment. He said yeah, but in that Rocky–New Jersey yeah way.

Finally, as he was being interviewed by one of the lead clinicians in the study, I raised the issue again. "Look," I said to her as nicely as I could, "given his profile — that he is asymptomatic, that there has not been new scarring, that he lives well, eats right, and gets plenty of exercise — let me ask a question. Would you give one of *your patients* — *not a research subject* — this drug?"

"Of course not," she said. "This is totally experimental. This drug combination isn't approved for standard treatment of hepatitis C." My father-in-law's eyes grew as big as pizza pies. It was the last time I heard anything from him or the doctor about "the new treatment." His liver has since improved on its own — dramatically even by the appraisal of his original specialist.

I tell this story not because I believe anyone could have done his or her job any better in this scenario, nor to run down the potential good of such an experiment for others in worse condition than my father-in-law, but merely to underscore how deeply the human impulse for a cure runs, and how willing we are to take the "cure" even when we have all the countervailing facts before us. It is a profound dynamic that can be exploited, both for good and for bad, and it is one that we should remember when assessing the ways of today's pharmaceutical companies. In short, we come preprogrammed to consume.

There is another reason behind our trust of pharma, one that is less obvious but, when stated fully, is as real as the Pfizer stock in Bob Dole's retirement portfolio: America has become a nation of pharmaceutical tribes. I refer to the emergence of three distinct audiences for treatment of chronic disease. The first we might call the Tribe of High-Performance Youth. This consists largely of children and adolescents who are medicated for depression, attention deficit disorder, bipolar disorder, and a range of other psychiatric and behavioral problems. Many of these children are rightly diagnosed; many are not. Many seem to benefit from these drugs, but we do not know the long-term consequences of treatment. The point is that they have become the most medicated generation of children in our history, and for one reason: their parents' completely understandable wish that they perform well in a society of ever increasing demands to perform well, nay, superbly.

The second group is the Middle-Years Tribe, or the Tribe of Productivity and Comfort, which consists of the middle-aged, those of us at the mid-to-late points in our careers as parents and/or earners. Our drugs range from antidepressants (Prozac, Paxil) to cholesterol reducers (Lipitor) to gastrointestinal agents (Prilosec) to painkillers (Vicodin) to libido enhancers (Viagra). The point of almost all of these drugs is to shore up our ability to produce more and better and to relieve discomfort, including the discomfort of having to watch what and how much we eat and drink and of sitting on our duff. There is nothing intrinsically wrong with that either, but the level of such medication is rising almost as fast as such levels among children, and it warrants our hardheaded consideration.

Lastly there is the Tribe of High-Performance Aging, of our elders. More than any other group, seniors take drugs not only to alleviate the discomfort of aging, but also to extend their lives. Who can begrudge anyone that? Yet as most of us who have cared for older loved ones know, the prescription drug cabinet can be a mixed blessing at best. Clinicians who specialize in the diseases of the elderly are increasingly concerned with the impact of extended pharmaceutical use. Note: That's *use*, not abuse or even overuse, that they're concerned about.

Of course, audiences for anything — drugs, movies, or even fast food — no longer just "happen" around a great performance or a great product; audiences, as any good marketing person will tell you, are created. And so it is with America's pharmaceutical tribes. Every one of them — and there are new ones every day — have a common birth mother, big pharma, which in recent years wholeheartedly embraced its new role as culture creator. Pharmaceutical companies do not sell drugs as much as they create awareness of "their" diseases. That is why you see giant demo booths for asthma spray at NASCAR races. As one marketing executive told me, "We are in the business of branding medical conditions."

This phenomenon isn't necessarily a bad thing, but it pays to note that the industry's ability to create mass consumer audiences is a fairly new phenomenon. Consider that the amount spent to advertise prescription drugs directly to consumers (called DTC) in 1980 was $2 million. In 2004, it was $4.35 billion and soaring. Twenty-five years ago, as this book will demonstrate, most drug company executives believed that DTC advertising not only wouldn't be good for business, but also, in the words of one pharma CEO, would be "one of the worst things that could happen to the doctor-patient relationship." Today, reality suggests that they were wrong about the business angle; DTC has been a gold mine. The number of Americans, annually, who request and receive a prescription for a specific drug after seeing a commercial for it is . . . 8.5 million. Once again, pretty soon, we're talking real money.

But do we know the full price for today's spiraling prescription drug culture? At one level, we know something about the immediate benefits of specific drugs. Pfizer's blockbuster, Lipitor, seems consistently to lower cholesterol levels and hence reduce cardiovascular *risks*, although there is still relatively little evidence that it prevents premature deaths, which might be something we want to know before we routinely prescribe it for everyone over fifty — itself a serious proposal by some of the world's top cardiologists. Similarly, Prilosec and its imitators seem to relieve the pain of the reflux disease GERD, although whether this class of drugs is worth the higher price, compared to its equally efficacious and low-priced predecessors, is debatable, and there is also growing concern that such gastrointestinal drugs might have worse long-term safety problems than originally advertised. Ritalin seems a good treatment for truly hyperactive children, but what does it do to an adolescent when he or she enters the experimental teen years? Ten million parents should want to know.

Yet these concerns, relatively speaking, are almost quibbles. The Big Question about all of these drugs might better be stated thus: Can our bodies, our pocketbooks, and our democratic institutions bear their cumulative cost? There are troubling signs that the answer is no.

First, there is the body. Consider the new pharmaceutical biography of just one key organ, the liver, charged with, among other things, disposing of toxins and making food into fuel. As the Food and Drug Administration (FDA), the American Medical Association (AMA), and every leading medical institution in this country and abroad has noted, liver damage, once rare, is now the leading reason for withdrawing a drug, usually a new drug, from the market. With more new drugs than ever before, the liver would have its lobes full even if other new trends didn't complicate matters further. The growing, lifelong "drug load" on the liver is one such concern — we now initiate prescriptions at a younger age than ever, take them for longer periods of time and often in greater amounts. There is also the growing tendency, particularly among the elderly, to use several daily drugs, which can combine to deliver a double whammy to the liver. Liver testing has itself become a boom industry in most large retirement communities. If that long-suffering organ could talk, one imagines it would say, perhaps in a pugnacious Brooklyn accent, "Hey, fella, I'm takin' a pastin' here, y'know what I'm sayin'?"

Add to this one other cheery number: There are more than 106,000 deaths a year from serious adverse drug reactions — from drugs that have been *properly* prescribed and taken. Considering that Vioxx alone may well have caused more than 100,000 deaths during its six-year run, the figure may be low. Even then, such reactions are now among the top ten causes of death in the United States. And that does not include deaths from overdose, drug abuse, or noncompliance.

Next there is the effect of prescriptions on the wallet, both collective and individual. National spending on prescription drugs, mainly via the Medicare law, will cost us trillions over the next decade; closer to home, pills are becoming the defining medical issue, perhaps more important than a doctor's visit or your next CAT scan. Their cost can break a senior's retirement fund — or send him running to the border for relief, not something most of our parents ever envisioned as part of their golden years.

Lastly comes government, for with the rise of pharmaceutical financial power has come a rise in its political clout. Its main tools are money, media power, and lobbying. Between 1996 and 2002, the industry spent half a billion dollars on lobbying, employing six hundred full-time lobbyists, among them twenty-four former members of Congress. Only recently did most Americans glimpse the extent of this power. Their peephole was the Medicare Prescription Drug Act, which the industry was able to rewrite to forbid the federal government from negotiating for lower drug prices — something citizens of every other industrialized democracy (and many undeveloped ones as well) take for granted. That the congressman who shepherded the bill is now the $2-million-a-year president of Pharmaceutical Research and Manufacturers of America (PhRMA), the industry's big lobbying group, takes no one by surprise.

The new pharma money also encourages regulatory permissiveness, both here and abroad. As a wide-ranging examination of the pharmaceutical industry in the British medical journal *The Lancet* recently concluded, "The present drug regulatory systems . . . are highly vulnerable to industrial capture, and permit the industry's scientific experts to have *extensive conflicts of interest* [my italics] while providing their expert advice." In other words, the FDA is too weak to stand up to the political machine of Eli Lilly, Pfizer, and Merck. Consider, for example, that the drug giant GlaxoSmithKline was cited by the FDA for deceptive and misleading advertising fourteen times between 1997 and 2001 but never fined. Or that between 1997 and 2001, the agency issued eighty-eight notices of violation for misleading print and TV ads·but could not levy even a single penalty.

One more statistic is in order here: of the 1,035 new drugs approved by the FDA between 1989 and 2000, more than one half represented "no significant clinical improvement" over older drugs. So why were they approved in the first place?

That last question begs others, the most important being: How did Americans become such enormous consumers of pharmaceuticals in the world, so much so that pills have become key transformers of both American bodies and American culture?

For the answer to that, we must first visit an engaging young man during the late years of Richard Nixon's tumultuous but ever enterprising White House . . .

Unbound

The Strange and Very American
Liberation of Big Pharma

THE MAN IN THE ARENA: WHY PHARMACEUTICAL
COMPANIES BECAME SO AGGRESSIVE

In the world of bureaucratic Washington, D.C., few if any possess the gravitas and smarts to get away with quoting Teddy Roosevelt. Lewis Engman, Richard Nixon's 1973 appointee as chairman of the powerful Federal Trade Commission (FTC), was one of the few. A Midwesterner with traditional Republican inclinations, Engman had "the gift," as one friend later put it — people simply wanted to be around him. He was a handsome man, with a broad brow and piercing dark eyes, and he was a social creature, stylishly dressed and coiffed and noticeable on the D.C. cocktail circuit, where he could be seen in the company of many of the president's closest advisers. Engman was a personable, if tightly wound, man as well, comfortable with business types and staff typists alike; when a young FTC appointee named Elizabeth Hanford (later Dole) had a minor accident and ended up in the emergency room on the day she was to be installed, Engman took his entire staff over to the hospital and swore her in while she was still in bed.

More importantly in a town of fiercely guarded opinions and fiefdoms, Lew Engman could take the heat of debate. He seemed to revel in it. Often he intentionally recruited lawyers with whom he did not agree. "The notion," a former staffer recalls, "was that the tension would produce the best resolution." That didn't mean Engman was thwarted very often; yes, he could be imperious and even arrogant, but "he was so personable and passionate that you *wanted* to agree with the guy."

Frustrated with the slow pace of getting anything done in D.C., Engman loved to invoke TR's famous "Man in the Arena" speech. "It is not the critic who counts; not the man who points out how the strong man stumbles or where the doer of deeds could have done better," he would quote, his brow furrowing. "The credit belongs to the man who is actually in the arena, whose face is marred by dust and sweat and blood, who strives valiantly, who errs and comes up short again and again, but who knows great enthusiasms . . . so that his place shall never be with those cold and timid souls who knew neither victory nor defeat."

It was an appropriate mission statement for a young man charged with running the FTC, which oversaw the business of the world's most powerful, if at the time troubled, economy. The FTC itself had grown increasingly controversial. For decades the commission had operated somewhat like a European or Japanese finance ministry, not simply policing industry's outright frauds and cons, but also regulating competition itself. The agencies under its purview, from the Civil Aviation Board (CAB) to the Interstate Commerce Commission (ICC), were so cozy with their respective industries that it was all but impossible for an upstart entrepreneur to compete. Traditionally the FTC chairman, in a tacit admission of the powerful regional political interests that had created that coziness, remained mute on the situation. "The policy was never to criticize another government agency," recalls Art Amolsch, who worked for Engman at the time and went on to become the foremost observer of the agency. "That's why the FTC was always known as the Old Lady of Pennsylvania Avenue. It was averse to almost any change and inclined to say no to anyone who dared suggest otherwise."

For a brief period in the late 1960s and early 1970s, responding to lawsuits and studies by Ralph Nader over everything from unsafe cars to overpriced drugs, the commission had gone on a proconsumer binge under Chairman Miles W. Kirkpatrick, and mainstream business types, the core of the imperiled president's political base, had railed against him during the 1972 election season. To calm them, in 1973 Nixon appointed Engman; he was supposed to "restore order." In other words, to put things back where they were before the Naderites inside the commission got out of control again.

But Nixon, and whoever had done the personnel file work, misjudged Engman's consumer credentials. Although he was a classic 100-percent-free-trade, procompetition Republican, Engman had developed a strong proconsumer bent. As *Time* magazine would later put it, Engman saw the world as a "Ralph Nader out of Adam Smith." You could best serve the consumer, he deduced, by opening up the marketplace.

With that in mind and the national economy in trouble — inflation was up and productivity was down — Engman went looking for ways to use the FTC's power to make the country more competitive and to make American life more affordable. Quickly he diagnosed a novel cancer on the nation's economic corpus: the regulatory agencies themselves. By making it so hard for small businesspeople to enter their respective industries, the CAB and ICC were hurting the consumer and inhibiting innovation, thereby retarding long-term economic growth and keeping prices unnaturally high. In a brilliant, landmark speech at the normally staid Financial Analysis Conference in 1974, he laid out his thesis: "Much of today's regulatory machinery does little more than shelter producers from the normal competitive consequences of lassitude and inefficiency . . . [it] has simply become perverted." As a result, "the consumer is paying plenty in the form of government-sanctioned price fixing." It was time, Engman said, to consider serious deregulation.

Engman also went after what he called "professional conspiracy." He sued the American Medical Association over its ban on physician advertising — something he believed deprived consumers of the ability to get the best doctor for the best price. He went after state medical societies for their bans on the advertisement of prescription drug and eyeglass prices. In fourteen months he filed thirty-four antitrust actions. "The consumer was always the bottom line for Lew," recalls Bob Lewis, who served on Engman's staff. "'Is this going to benefit the consumer?' That was always the question he asked at the end of the debate about anything."

By the time he left the FTC in 1977, when a Democratic administration was about to take office, Engman had succeeded in making deregulation a mainstream Republican goal. At age forty-two, he was a GOP legend.

And so it was hardly surprising that, in the fall of 1980, with a new president named Ronald Reagan onboard who was committed to getting government out of every aspect of American life, Engman would again be sought for his leadership skills. This time the organization in need of help was the Pharmaceutical Manufacturer Associations. The PMA represented the nation's biggest brand-name drug makers, who were often referred to simply as "big pharma" or simply "pharma." (The organization itself formally changed its name to the Pharmaceutical Research and Manufacturers of America, PhRMA, in 1994.) The PMA believed that the industry was in a crisis, suffering from increasing costs, slipping sales, foreign competition, and government over-regulation. It was a crisis so severe as to provoke pharma CEOs to wonder out loud "whether there will even be a U.S. pharmaceuticals industry in twenty years." Then again, just about every major industry wondered something like that in the early 1980s, when it was widely believed that Japan was doing to U.S. industry what it had failed to do with bombs thirty-five years earlier.

Some, if not most, of pharma's immediate crisis was of its own making, although this was not something most drug CEOs would admit. As a group and individually, they had simply failed to invest in new drug sciences and drug development. Instead, they had relied on (and indeed encouraged) the FDA's lack of a generic-drug approval process, giving pharmaceutical companies de facto monopolies — and huge profit margins — on many widely used drugs. This state of affairs had provoked a legal backlash of its own; district courts from New York to California were actively contemplating, and in some cases ruling, that many traditional pharmaceutical patents were invalid. The Supreme Court itself had grown hostile to the very notion of patents. In the pharma executive suite of the time, there was only one word for that: shock.

Yet some pharma problems were largely out of the industry's direct control. America in the late 1970s and early 1980s was going through one of its cyclical periods of what might be dubbed pharmaceutical stoicism. As a percentage of annual health expenditures, the Rx share was actually shrinking. And while cocaine might be hip, prescription drugs were uncool on a number of levels. On the cultural plane, drug makers were the domain of the blue-chip world, with which the baby boom had yet to fall in love. The growing alternative-medicine movement, with its reliance on herbs and vitamins, appealed to a generation concerned with what was natural. The movie version of *One Flew Over the Cuckoo's Nest* rekindled old suspicions about psychiatric medications, one of the industry's most profitable monopolies. News stories about abuse of Valium, one of the most profitable postwar drugs, led to its reclassification as a controlled substance in 1978, making it harder to prescribe. There were scares over new heart medications and horror stories about pharmaceutical-industry negligence, and a new generation of ambitious politicians had no qualms about capitalizing on such fears. When a young congressman named Albert Gore learned from a staffer that a Pfizer attorney had made an off-the-cuff remark about how expensive it was to monitor the adverse events of one of his products ("What, are we supposed to schlep all over the world just to track down one goddamn side effect?" the attorney had sputtered), Gore promptly publicized the incident. Abroad and in D.C., big pharma was, more than ever, big fair game.

Worse from the point of view of pharmaceutical CEOs were attitudes and trends among young physicians and medical students. Many of them were deeply suspicious of the business end of medicine. Some of their attitudes grew from social activism by med students in the early 1970s, who were concerned with overmedication and polypharmacy. (Overmedication is the unnecessary use of medications in general; polypharmacy is the simultaneous use of several medications to treat one or more conditions.) The concern was deepest among young psychiatrists. "In our day, it was almost an aesthetic thing to be against polypharmacy," recalls one. "It was more beautiful if you could do it with just one or two pills." Many believed that growing rates of polypharmacy were fueled by pharma promotional activities, like giving out free samples and stethoscopes. "At national meetings, the idea we talked about was to reject the goodies," recalls Dr. Terry Kupers, who was head of the Medical Committee for Human Rights in the 1970s. "[Pharma sales representatives] would show up at grand rounds, and we would confront them and turn down the goodies. We also went to our intern meetings within our institutions and told our supervisors that we did not want [the reps] on grand rounds. It was happening at enlightened medical schools around the country. We did it as a statement."

The statement registered in establishment realms, a further worry to pharma, when, in 1978, a number of influential medical journals began to consider banning prescription drug ads in their pages. As Steve Conafay, then a lobbyist for Pfizer, recalls, "There was definitely the feeling that the industry was under attack and that something big had to be done." Donald Rumsfeld, then the CEO of G. D. Searle, Inc., makers of a wide variety of drugs and chemicals, summed up the general attitude when, upon greeting FDA Commissioner Donald Kennedy, he "sat down across from me," recalls Kennedy, "slumped a little, and said, 'What are we doing wrong?'"

With Reaganism ascendant, the question quickly turned into: What is the government doing wrong? For Engman, now ensconced in PMA's head office, the question should have been: What can I wring out of the new political reality — Reagan's pronounced antiregulatory bent — that will directly benefit my membership, the nation's brand-name drug makers? Certainly many of his members were clamoring for a preemptive strike, with several advocating an assault on the FDA and its much-hated efficacy requirements. (Congress had passed a law in 1962, known as the Kefauver Amendments, changing the Food and Drug Act and mandating that makers of new drugs prove not just that their products were safe, but that they actually worked.) The chief of research at Pfizer, then as now one of the more politically active pharmaceutical companies, had been railing against the efficacy rules for years, saying they got in the way of delivering good new drugs.

But Engman didn't think that way. He wasn't interested in deregulation for deregulation's sake. Perhaps it was that consumer bug, or perhaps it was his heady experience as leader of an agency that served "the public." Whatever the exact source of Engman's reservations, his eventual choice of legislative priorities finally came down to one issue: patent restoration. The subject had bubbled under the surface of FDA-industry relations for years. Simply put, the industry believed that the FDA was eating up the length of its patents, and profits, because of its slowness in processing new drug applications. Companies with a new discovery had to file for a patent as soon as possible, to establish ownership of the idea, but then had to wait years for approval. By the time the drug was approved, the company might have as little as half the original seventeen years of patent life usually guaranteed to innovators. That led to higher prices, longer waits for new drugs, and a general disincentive to invest in new medications. It was true that the studies proving the case for patent restoration — for laws that would give pharma additional compensatory patent time — were weak and inconclusive, but the essence of the industry argument struck a nerve with Engman: here again was a case of overregulation hurting the economy of the nation and depriving the consumer of an improved product.

What should Engman's PMA do? Sometime during the fall of 1980, he got an idea. He would use his old political contacts to shepherd legislation to extend pharmaceutical patents, adding up to seven years of exclusive marketing time for new drugs that had taken too long to get through the FDA approval process.

For a while, all of the old Engman magic seemed to work. He circulated studies showing exactly how industry suffered from FDA bureaucracy — and how few new important drugs made it through the system. He lined up experts from leading medical schools to testify on the subject before Congress. By late 1982, he had managed to push the political process as well. A bill extending patent life was passed by the Senate and referred to the House for an expedited vote.

Yet the world — and particularly Washington, D.C. — does not lie under the spell of magic for long, and Engman's bill went down to unexpected defeat. One reason was the weather; a dense winter storm had settled over Foggy Bottom on the morning of the vote, delaying the arrival of several key supporters. Then there was another, less natural phenomenon: a man named Henry Waxman.

Waxman, a short, balding, mustachioed man who represented the Westside of Los Angeles, was the quintessential manifestation of the new post-Vietnam liberal legislator. In just nine years he had risen from relative obscurity to the chairmanship of the powerful Subcommittee on Health and Environment of the House Energy and Commerce Committee. This ascent he accomplished via the unabashed use of a political action committee, by which he funded the campaigns of like-minded fellow Democrats, who would then support his nomination to important committees. Perhaps more importantly, Waxman was a single-focus legislator by design, rather than by circumstance. "I recall him coming up to me at a fundraiser very early is his career and telling me he had found the key to his political life," one longtime supporter remembered. "He said, 'It's health. Who can be against health?'" If Waxman's concern seemed calculated, it was also genuine. Some of Waxman's earliest supporters were older, less affluent Westsiders who were constantly kvetching to him about the price of prescription drugs.

"There was no way that Henry was going to give the industry seven more years of protected profits," says Bill Corr, then head of Waxman's committee staff. "The more we looked at Engman's so-called studies, the more we saw something else. For their most profitable drugs, the brand-name companies had actually received a substantial — sometimes lengthy — period of monopoly patent protection."

There was another less tangible but, in the end, highly potent factor at play in Waxman's position as well: the belief that many of the brand-name pharma CEOs were anti-Semitic. Waxman had arrived at that conclusion after a series of initial meetings with the CEOs and their representatives. "Whenever they talked about the generics guys, the word they like to use the most was 'parasite,'" Waxman recalls. "Then they would talk about how greedy they were, how they throve off of the back of people who did the real work. I thought it was anti-Semitic. You could feel it. They were so disdainful, these New Jersey country club types."

Waxman's anti–brand name inclinations were further inflamed by another political bomb-thrower, a man named Bill Haddad. Haddad was the head of the Generic Pharmaceutical Industry Association (GPIA) and the owner of a small copycat drug company, but he was no industry hack. He had a long, distinguished (if eclectic) liberal heritage dating back to his days on the staff of Senator Estes Kefauver, the author of the important 1962 efficacy amendments. It was through Kefauver that Haddad picked up the emotional component of his anti–brand name jihad, the rhetoric of which often included such unconventional words as "liars" and "immoral" to describe his opponents. As Haddad saw it, it was the industry's intransigence on such issues as generics and open pricing that had pushed Kefauver over the edge physically, eventually causing his death from a heart attack in 1963. (Kefauver's legislation had been rewritten at the last minute behind his back by Kennedy administration staffers and brand-name lobbyists, who deleted the senator's beloved generics provisions.) Haddad loved to tell the story of how he had visited Kefauver's grave in the rain and swore: "I'll get those bastards, senator."

For two decades, he had done just that, first through a series of journalistic exposés (Haddad had extensive family media connections and earlier had won a Pulitzer Prize for a series on price fixing in the antibiotics industry), then, in the 1970s, through his work in the New York state legislature. There, as a staff member with subpoena power, he had forced the brand-name firms to disclose which drugs were off patent. He then put together a powerful case against then prevalent anti-generic-substitution laws, which pharma executives had pushed through state legislatures across the country, thus making the prescribing of generics almost impossible. After New York repealed its antigeneric laws, Haddad put together a how-to kit for repeal and sent it out to "every ambitious young state legislator across the country." Within a few years every such law in the country had been wiped from the books.

But Haddad's biggest beef with the industry — and the FDA — had provoked little in the way of action. By 1982 there was still no workable economic method for getting a generic drug approved even after a patent ran out. That was because the FDA still required any maker of a generic version of a brand-name drug to undertake the same lengthy, costly, and sometimes dangerous series of clinical trials to prove its product was safe and efficacious. Technically, this process was totally unnecessary. Time-proven methods of reverse engineering, along with sophisticated ways of assaying copycat compounds, could assure that any generic was biologically equivalent. "It was totally immoral to insist that the generic maker do all that again," Haddad argued. "But they don't care . . . they don't care about the senior citizens, they don't care about the poor single mother, they don't care . . ." Many inside the FDA agreed, but the political power of the PMA, along with institutional inertia, cowardice, and plain old bureaucratic ass-covering had precluded any meaningful reform.

Then, in mid-1982, just as the PMA and Engman were using a new, ostensibly "independent" study to convince Congress that patent life had been dramatically shortened by FDA red tape, Haddad got a letter from a woman in Florida, a statistician who claimed she had been an author of the supposedly independent study. "She said that not only had the numbers for the study been prepared for her by the industry, but that the brand names had paid for the study and then insisted that it be presented as 'independent.'" Haddad used the disclosure to stir up discontented seniors in two Miami Beach districts, who in turn "drove their congressman crazy" about why patent restoration was wrong, not to mention political suicide. Using Haddad's activism to mobilize opposition votes and Al Gore's willingness to vilify the industry in general, Waxman defeated Engman's patent-extension legislation.

For a time following his defeat, Engman worked on a number of other industry-relief efforts. Certainly the time was still right for anything that offered a way to make the nation more competitive. Congress had passed the Bayh-Dole Act in 1981, which made it easier for the industry to use research discoveries that originated in publicly funded laboratories. For pharma, that opened up a wide range of lucrative partnerships with researchers at the National Institutes of Health (NIH), where scientists were making breakthroughs in developing new molecules that could treat everything from heart disease to depression. The law also made it possible for government researchers to accept consulting fees from pharmaceutical companies.

This opening-up process — in essence doing away with old church-state separations that favored institutional or scientific independence over commerce of almost any kind — was the subject of a lengthy inquiry from some of the nation's leading experts in pharmacology and drug regulation, who were joined by Engman. Commenced in the late 1970s under Tulane University's Dr. Gilbert McMahon, the Commission on the Federal Drug Approval Process was originally created as an evenhanded, fact-finding mission to discern whether many of the industry's complaints about the FDA were justified. Under Reagan, it essentially became an industry organ, funded not by the government but — under the guise of budgetary efficiency — by private interests and philanthropists in tune with the president's deregulatory impulses. As a result, the commission's official discussions about opening up the FDA took place off the record and out of media view at a Virginia resort owned by a friend of the president.

By the time the commission presented its report in late 1982, almost every discordant (i.e., anti–brand name) note had been tuned out. Instead, what Congress heard was a venerable choir of scientific voices demanding that the FDA cut the red tape and speed up approvals. The commission then presented Congress with its list of recommendations, many of which would eventually make it into the law books. Instead of requiring extensive, multiple studies for approval, the commission asked that "effectiveness should be found to have been demonstrated either by two — or, when appropriate, one — adequately designed and well-controlled studies." Foreign studies should also be admissible and given equal weight with domestic studies, even if the populations were different. The commission also advised lifting stodgy old conflict-of-interest restrictions that barred the use of industry-paid experts in FDA advisory committee meetings. Lastly, "the FDA should provide guidance to its staff to encourage all review personnel to conduct timely, forthright, and even-handed discussions with sponsors that arise at any time during the review process."

"That last one was the one that really mattered, long-term," says Jonah Shacknai, then a commission staff member and now the president of Millennium Pharmaceuticals. "The real importance of the recommendations was a closer relationship between FDA and manufacturers. It used to be a solid Chinese wall. Now it had good windows in it."

But "good windows" into a regulatory agency were not what Lew Engman had in mind. He had patent reform in mind. True, there was now a little bit of obsession at work — "he could get very wound up about it" — yet as he listened to Waxman and Haddad talk, there were also other legitimate pinpricks on his conscience. What if Haddad was right? What if the PMA was on the wrong side of history? After all, in a recent district court ruling, *Bolar v. Roche*, a Brooklyn judge had ruled that it was not an infringement of a patent if a generics maker used a patented drug for experimental purposes in preparation for a regulatory hearing. That meant that more generics were inevitable. It would become known as the Bolar exemption.

There was also troubling momentum on the Hill. Waxman had introduced new legislation that would make it easier for generics to get approval — and with no provision for patent term restoration for the brand-name companies at all. Waxman had, in fact, shifted the entire debate. Now the "greedy" ones were the brand-name companies — something he repeated with nauseating regularity any time the media tuned in. And there was the quintessential Engman worry: Was the PMA's opposition to a faster generics process — an abbreviated new drug application (ANDA) — not all that different from the FTC countenancing the Civil Aviation Board's coziness with industry? Weren't all those FDA regulations requiring duplicate testing another form of overregulation that hurt the economy and the consumer? What if Haddad was morally right?

Slowly, Engman started to talk about the whole issue differently, recalls Bob Smith, one of his closer staff aides at the PMA. "The companies are basically using human testing to protect the pill patents," he recalls Engman saying one day. It wasn't the first time anyone had put it quite that way, but it was the first time the head of the PMA had, or at least the first time one had done so out loud. Not long after, Engman assigned his lead counsel to begin negotiations with Haddad and Waxman's staff to cut a deal: the PMA would trade its opposition to generics for a guarantee of patent term restoration. A deal was struck with Waxman's staff. It included the Bolar exemption, thus putting into the law books what had only recently been rendered by a district court. Generic companies could now use formerly protected brand-name compounds to develop their low-price alternatives.

Immediately, a small but loud group of pharma CEOs called for Engman to abandon the deal. "I thought Lew had gone out of his tree," says Irwin Lerner, then the head of Hoffmann-LaRoche, which made Valium. "He was embarrassed by it, I could tell. But he was also arrogant about it. He wasn't going to back off the deal. His attitude was, 'Who the hell are these guys around the table telling me what to do?' He thought he was still the head of the FTC."

"All of the sudden, these guys who had been for the deal started freaking out," recalls Bob Smith. "All of a sudden, everyone had an exception — What about my Valium? What about my Inderal? They were all afraid that one company would get an advantage the other would not. Lew wasn't totally surprised by it, but he was determined to live up to his deal with Waxman."

Joe Williams, then the chairman of the PMA board and the

head of Parke-Davis, was furious. He asked for Engman's resignation. The man in the arena was fired.

To derail the new bill, Williams and Lerner turned to an unexpected source, a man named Gerry Mossinghoff. Tall, owlish, and charming in an old-school sort of way, Mossinghoff was the U.S. commissioner of patents and trademarks. As such, he was committed to traditional patent law, and barely an official phrase passed his lips without Mossinghoff uttering something about "classic, hornbook patent law," referring to the nineteenth-century case books that informed his views. He was also a textbook Reaganite, inclined to look unfavorably at regulatory or legislative limits on patent life. He had helped the president establish and populate a new, conservative patent court. Just who "requested" that he get involved and testify before Congress on the pro–brand name side is unclear, and there were recriminations all around. It was an unusual position for a paid public servant to be in.

But it was too late. Bill Haddad had made sure that the legislation would not get sabotaged by going directly to the congressman most likely to do so: Senator Orrin Hatch of Utah. Socially and fiscally conservative, Hatch was a supporter of pharma, but he had a pronounced populist streak as well. He had a yearning to transcend his narrow reputation as a conservative firebrand. To exploit that, Haddad hired Hatch's longtime chief of staff, who had just gone into private practice as a lobbyist, to convince his old boss to come onboard. Here was a great opportunity to expand and broaden his image, and, as Hatch was told, "generics seemed to be the right thing to do" to boot. Hatch agreed. The Waxman bill became Hatch-Waxman — the order of the names reflecting not effort but clout — and was signed that fall.

The reaction in big pharma's executive suites was startlingly clear and everywhere evident. There was now a new reality in the business, and that new reality was fear — fear of not exploiting drugs fast enough and hard enough before generic competition eroded profits. And there was only one way to do that: get more new drugs approved faster and find new ways to milk them once they were approved.

To help ease the political way, the brand-name companies

hired a new PMA president. His name was Gerry Mossinghoff. As Roche's Irv Lerner said, "He had all the tickets we could possibly want."

THE MAN IN THE MIDDLE: HOW PHARMA
REINVENTED PATIENTS AND THE FDA

One of the things that Roche's Irv Lerner and Parke-Davis's Joe Williams liked about Gerry Mossinghoff — besides the former patent commissioner's simpatico view of patent law and his many useful governmental connections — was his vision of federal regulatory agencies. "About that, he was fresh," recalls Williams. Unlike Lew Engman, who saw in the regulatory agencies some kind of compact between the public and its leaders, Gerry Mossinghoff discerned unfulfilled commercial promise. Period. As a bona fide Reaganite, he viewed regulatory bodies as impediments to industrial competitiveness — not because they regulated, but because they regulated inefficiently. Mossinghoff witnessed the phenomenon firsthand when the president appointed him commissioner to the United States Patent and Trademark Office (USPTO) in 1980. "I remember coming to headquarters, and someone taking me over to the Crystal City offices, where there were basically three floors of unopened mail!" As Mossinghoff saw it, in all that mail lay the possible seeds of countless inventions that could revive the national economy.

Mossinghoff's solution was to remake the USPTO's relationship with business into one of client and service provider. To that end, he instituted the concept of user fees; as he reasoned, just as a businessman might pay a lawyer to review a risky new venture, so should a corporation with a new patent application be allowed to pay for its expedited review by the government. True, there were some inherent contradictions in the very notion of "government user" fees. After all, companies were required by law to submit to the USPTO if they wanted a patent, and the government (a.k.a. taxpayers) employed legions of reviewers that were supposed to evaluate each patent *objectively* and with an eye not just for the private gain, but for the public gain as well.

But Mossinghoff was not concerned with such old-line preoccupations. He was a pragmatist, and, because of his closeness to Malcolm Baldridge, one of the president's most trusted economic advisers, he could get things done. And so he did: In short order, Mossinghoff's user fees became a huge success story. By the time he left the USPTO for the PMA, the period a company had to wait before receiving a patent shrunk from more than three years to fewer than eighteen months.

Almost as soon as he landed at the PMA, Mossinghoff began talking user fees again. He thought the industry needed more of "a client–service provider relationship" with the FDA. It was an idea that appealed to the more progressive CEOs within big pharma. So one day in early 1985, Irv Lerner and Joe Williams arranged a meeting with Mossinghoff to learn just how that might happen. For both executives, it was a revelatory tutelage. As their new PMA president laid it out, slow review times at the FDA had nothing to do with the agency being "hostile" to new drugs. The holdup was about money — or, in governmental terms, "low budgetary allocations for review staff." As a result, agency reviewers — safety experts, epidemiologists, chemistry analysts, study evaluators — were chronically behind schedule. Mossinghoff proposed that pharma companies address that real need by paying fees to the agency whenever they filed new drug applications, or NDAs. He also rubbed a raw spot. "I told them, 'Look, getting new drugs approved would be a key in the battle against the lost profits due to new generics.'" Suddenly a thousand-watt bulb lit up. As Lerner recalls, "I thought, Wow, what would it be worth if we could pay a fee and get a faster review?"

Yet as much sense as user fees for faster FDA review made to Lerner, it was a disaster when he and Mossinghoff presented the concept to the assembled PMA board in 1986. "They thought I was some kind of left-wing liberal," Lerner recalls. "Merck and Pfizer hated it. They viewed it as just another tax." In their rejection, however, Mossinghoff discerned more than a small institutional setback. Pharma, he became convinced, was simply out of touch — out of touch with regulatory realities, out of touch with doctors, who wrote prescriptions, and, perhaps most troublingly, out of touch with patients, the people who were, after all, the end consumers of their labor. As Bob Allnutt, his chief of staff, re-called, "When we got to the PMA, it was startlingly clear that it did not have any relationships with anybody — barely with the AMA! Among the major patient groups, no one ever called us."

Yet by the mid-1980s, many understood that, among patients and patient organizations alike, a great generational revolution had commenced. At its proverbial red-hot center were activists concerned with the mounting devastation of AIDS. The disease and the reaction to it had caught the industry completely off-guard, recalls John Peck, a consultant to the PMA in the early 1990s. "I recall one day getting a phone call from the head of a di-vision of one of the biggest pharma companies, and him telling me how he had been so proud that his company had decided to become proactive and call in AIDS patient groups and tell them what they were doing," says Peck. "Well, the patients had looked across the table at them and said, 'Fine, we like what you are do-ing. By the way, we have a copy of your research protocol and we'd like to talk to you about that.' The company was shocked. They had never seen patient organizations with that kind of savvy and network."

The new assertiveness was hardly limited to AIDS activists. As baby boomers aged, so did their demand for state-of-the-art medical information. And it wasn't just information they were seeking. Managed care, and its rising encroachments on what they once considered an entitlement, was forcing boomers to ar-ticulate their medical rights, which they had not had to do be-fore. In a sense, an entire generation was finding and forging a new medical identity. "A huge psychographic was blowing up," says Peck. "To Gerry Mossinghoff, the writing was on the wall — you better get with this and find a way to lead."

To do so, Mossinghoff quietly set up a new organization called the Healthcare Quality Alliance, which he underwrote and in-stalled in a corner of the PMA's headquarters. The alliance's charge was to coordinate and support a wide range of new and traditional patient organizations, from the American Diabetes Association to the American Cancer Society, and then find areas where "our interests are synonymous with theirs," as one staff member put it. At first the new organization simply lobbied for increased spending on basic medical science at the NIH, using patient groups and individuals to make the case on the Hill. Yet as word of the new symbiosis, or "synonymous interests," spread — as did word of the PMA's largesse — the alliance was used for other, more tangible and more immediate concerns. As Joe Isaacs, a staffer at the National Health Council who worked closely with the PMA at the time, recalls, "We basically created the disease-of-the-month club." Through the alliance, the PMA would underwrite what it called "educational opportunities for members of Congress," sending patients and physicians armed with state-of-the-art information about breakthrough medications to the Hill.

There were almost immediate returns on the investment. When Medicare balked at paying for expensive new beta-blocking drugs, the alliance would marshal a phalanx of patients to visit the Hill en masse. If there was resistance at the FDA to approving, say, new allergy and asthma drugs, patients would be sent off bearing data that showed that allergies, for example, were the number one reason for lost school days, essentially making an economic argument for the drug that might not be appreciated at those stodgy FDA advisory meetings. What about new legislation to expedite review and approval of expensive AIDS drugs? Again, the PMA could now call on a wide range of gay political action groups to buttonhole lawmakers. At bottom, the alliance became a way to put a human face on any pharmacomedical demand — and if the demand happened to further pharma goals, so much the better.

New synergies bred newer synergies. It soon became clear that the alliance was exerting an enterprising influence on the patient organizations themselves. "It pushed a lot of our members to see that they could also be more assertive at the FDA," says Isaacs. "They could also have a voice in the drug approval process," mainly through testifying at scientific advisory meetings, which often give the key thumbs-up or -down on a new drug. Mossinghoff encouraged the trend. He realized that such testimony would be effective and forthcoming at the right time — when any given NDA was in trouble — if and only if he built strong relations with patient groups early in the approval process. If he didn't, he would leave himself open to the charge of opportunism.

To that end, he encouraged individual pharmaceutical companies to bring patient groups to their plants and show them what they were doing in their R&D departments, illustrating firsthand why drugs cost so much. "That really helped build a trusting relationship between the patient groups and pharma," says Myrl Weinberg, then head of the National Health Council. "So when individual pharma companies knew they were having trouble with a drug at FDA they would go to the groups ahead of time and brief them about what it might be appropriate to say in an advisory meeting. That was new." By the early 1990s, Mossinghoff had succeeded in repairing pharma's connections to patients and patient groups, in the process turning old-fashioned patient relations into powerful new ways of moving pharma's political and financial agenda forward.

No one seemed more attuned to that transformation than Senator Edward Kennedy, traditionally a huge pharma enemy. He, like Waxman, had built much of his political identity around the notion that, because he was always loudly against big pharma, he was always for the consumer, which meant that you should vote for him and not PfizerSatanGOP man. Now, it seemed, the tables were turned. Somehow pharma, and not traditional liberal health-care warriors, was becoming a standard-bearer for patients, who, of course, were also voters. The psychographic had lurched right. It hurt doubly that many of these propharma voters were gay voters, whose rights and interests had once been the sole domain of the liberal establishment. Kennedy was also getting a propharma message from his own constituents in Massachusetts's surging biotech industry, many of whom were pharma-based. Why, even the new FDA commissioner, a young physician named David Kessler whom Kennedy liked for his antitobacco rants, seemed open to industry initiatives.

As Mossinghoff and his closest aides saw it, if there was ever a time to persuade his pharma colleagues to sign on to user fees for NDAs, this was it. He and Irv Lerner cooked up a slogan to go with the legislative campaign. "We were always saying, 'An educated FDA reviewer is our best customer,'" Lerner recalls. "That drove it home to the CEOs that this was an opportunity, not just another government fee or tax." To the objection that user fees might end up merely funding other, nonpharma departments of the FDA, Mossinghoff made sure the new legislation mandated that all user fees be strictly dedicated to hiring and supporting drug reviewers. What if review times didn't shorten — wouldn't that mean that the companies would be stuck with fees *and* the same old delays? To that Mossinghoff responded with what many to this day believe was a stroke of genius, a stroke that forever changed the culture of the FDA. "I said, 'Why don't we just say that the law has to be renewed every five years and that the FDA commissioner should be required, just like a CEO, to show progress toward the goal of reducing review time or the agency will not get the fees anymore?'"

This tack immediately appealed to the new FDA chief, Kessler, because it solved an age-old political problem at the agency: whenever an FDA commissioner dared to inquire why review times of NDAs were slow, he was immediately accused of circumventing the process, or, worse, running some secret agenda for pharma and its minions. As Bob Allnutt put it, "For the first time, the FDA chief had legitimate cover to put the heat on reviewers for at least a discussion on why an NDA was not moving forward." The Prescription Drug User Fee Act, or PDUFA, passed in 1992 with relatively little public debate. Its impact was swift and dramatic and generally considered positive.

There were, however, some fairly gaping holes in the legislation, and they soon set a number of serious insiders to worrying. By far the biggest concern was the issue of pharmacovigilance, a big word with a very simple meaning: the monitoring of drugs *after* they have been approved for sale. Traditionally the FDA had handled that through a scantily funded department that depended on voluntary reporting of safety problems from doctors, patients, and drug companies. Everyone knew that the system was weak, with only 10 percent of total adverse events being reported. Yet even though the PDUFA would clearly result in dozens of new drugs entering the marketplace, the law provided no new money for increased safety surveillance. Although the agency tried to compensate by requiring companies to perform postmarketing studies, almost none of them complied, believing that the requirement would eventually be eliminated.

There was, in fact, a growing truculence by the companies in general to meet with FDA reviewers if that meant dealing with anything negative, or "nonproductive." The arrogance was palpable, a far cry from Donald Rumsfeld's "What are we doing wrong?" lament of a decade or so earlier. In 1992, after withdrawal of its drug Omniflox, officials from Abbott Laboratories simply refused to show up and meet with FDA safety people. At a scientific advisory meeting on using the drug tamoxifen for breast cancer, according to a longtime observer, "You could read between the lines that the reviewers were just screaming that the companies were not providing all the information." This standoff persisted because only Congress — not the FDA — has the subpoena power to compel companies to supply *all* data. And ever since the PDUFA, congressional interest in such oversight "has completely dried up," says the same observer. "Are they too busy? Do they not have the technical resources? I don't know."

Perhaps just as troubling were reports coming from inside the FDA. Larry Sasich of Public Citizen, a longtime pharma and FDA watchdog group, was particularly worried by what he was hearing at the level of FDA scientific advisory committee meetings, which he had followed for thirty years. Patient testimony was twisting the normally staid and careful process. "A marketing person would tell you that people would rather hear miracles than horror stories, and we saw that the scientists were no different," Sasich says. One of the worst examples was a series of hearings prior to the approval of Lotronex, a drug for irritable bowel syndrome that the advisory panel approved but which was eventually pulled for safety reasons. "Scientists were shown the horrors but did not pay attention to it." They were deflected from it by the patient-witnesses' more emotional pleas. There were also problems with the FDA reviewers themselves. Despite the addition of user fees to their budgets, the pressure for them to produce increased even more so. By 1997, a survey of all medical officers, including the head of the agency's Center for Drug Evaluation, indicated that the PDUFA had created "a sweatshop atmosphere."

Nevertheless, despite these concerns, the PDUFA was renewed in 1997 with great fanfare. By then two things were clear. One was that Gerry Mossinghoff's dream of a clientized FDA had come true. New drug approvals were being issued in unprecedented numbers, and review times were at historic lows. There were important new drugs on the market for AIDS, cancer, heart disease, and stroke. And there was a vast new world of drugs for chronic diseases, from depression to something called gastroesophageal reflux disease (GERD), once known as heartburn. As the January 1997 issue of the pharma trade magazine *Scrips* noted, more pharmaceutical companies chose the United States for the introduction of their new drugs into market than any other country in the world. As Jeff Bloom, the head of the influential Patients' Coalition, put it in congressional testimony that year, "It clearly follows, then, that the FDA must be doing something right." Mossinghoff was triumphant.

"TO PUSH THE PHYSICIAN'S ARM": HOW PILLS LEARNED TO TALK

Getting the FDA into approval mode was a near Olympian victory for the Gerry Mossinghoffs and Irv Lerners of the world. Why, it was as if one had turned on the tap of an ancient well that no one expected would ever produce again and then, *swoosh*, a gusher spouted. But it was *near* Olympian. To clinch the gold, one had to figure out the next part of the commercial equation: what to do with all those pills? After all, it was one thing to get new drugs approved, but it was quite another to get people to buy them.

While the drug approval system was changing, the drug distribution system — the manner in which people got drugs — was not. Compared to the full-on spigot at the FDA, the pipeline to the patient was a bottleneck: every drug dispensed and paid for at the pharmacy was the end result of a long and slow process of convincing individual physicians to take a chance on a new treatment. Worse, the bottleneck was thin. Eighty percent of all prescriptions in the United States were issued via a mere 400,000 physicians. And, to torment the metaphor, the bottle was of the ketchup variety: sometimes it could take two or three years to get those physicians to "write" a new drug, even if it was a great new drug. That took a lot of costly bottle thumping. Two or three years? Given the imperatives of impending generic competition, such was a luxury few could afford, particularly those in the anxious, post–Hatch-Waxman executive suite of big pharma.

Yet even by the mid-1980s, when consumer advertising of everything from food to electronics soared far beyond any previous limits, the idea of selling prescription drugs directly to patients via TV or radio was anathema to most mainstream pharmaceutical executives. Some of their hesitation was generational. Many of these men (and they were all men) had scientific or medical backgrounds, and the thought of advertising a drug to anyone but a physician — and even then in very low-key ways — was vulgar. How could they ever explain that to the many medical men on their corporate boards? And for the rare executive bold enough to break with the ranks, there were two jet-cooling horror stories, one medical, one political, that almost always halted the discussion dead in its tracks.

The medical caveat came via Eli Lilly, which in the early 1980s introduced a novel arthritis drug named Oraflex. To distinguish it from others in a deeply competitive category, young executives in Lilly's marketing department decided on a new tack. In the past, companies might send out information kits to medical journals, trying to drum up some free trade coverage. But only physicians who actually flipped through their weekly periodicals saw those. Lilly's Oraflex team decided to expand the concept: why not send the kits out to thousands of mainstream press outlets, including TV and radio, perhaps pushing the notion (albeit technically unproven) that Oraflex actually healed tissues and hence might "cure" arthritis? Their strategy, which today might be considered comically tame, was radical for its day and quickly generated enormous media attention. The result: Lilly sold an unprecedented half a million prescriptions of Oraflex in its first fourteen weeks on the market. Unfortunately, the drug turned out to be a potent liver and kidney toxin, causing fifty deaths before it was eventually pulled from the market in 1983. It was often cited, long and loudly, in any discussion about direct-to-consumer advertising.

The political caveat, also from the early 1980s, grew out of the experience of one Dr. Arthur Hull Hayes, President Reagan's first nominee to head the FDA. A lanky, bookish man with a substantial background in clinical pharmacology (the study of how drugs work in a therapeutic, as opposed to experimental, setting), Hayes was generally regarded as a political moderate. He had once worked as a consultant to Roche, but he also had deep links to the academic and scientific community. He liked to talk about how he might speed up the drug approval process, but he was a stickler for details. And there was one thing that most seemed to preoccupy Hayes: the subject of "patient information." Ever since coming to the FDA, he had gotten an earful from the Reagan cabinet about new regulations, promulgated under Hayes's liberal predecessor, Dr. Jere Goyan, requiring drug makers to provide a "patient information insert" with every prescription. Reagan's deregulation-minded cabinet hated the idea, and saw it as one more example of too much government. Hayes was instructed by the White House to get rid of the program, and he did.

But in the process of wrestling with that issue, Hayes quietly became a convert to the notion of direct-to-consumer (DTC) prescription drug advertising. It wasn't a big stretch for him; unlike so many academics, not to mention FDA careerists, Hayes arrived unburdened by elitist opposition to advertising in general. Both his mother and father were employed in the industry — his father eventually became president of CBS Radio — and one summer young Arthur, as a student, worked in the mailroom of the ad giant McCann Erickson. As far as he was concerned, ad people were "among the most creative and knowledgeable people to be found anywhere in our society," and advertising was simply one part of the great American system, inexorably connected to the process of innovation and change and betterment. Opposing DTC, Hayes came to believe, simply put the industry and the government on the wrong side of history: Why, just look at the consumer movement, he said. That wasn't going away. People wanted to know more about what they were buying. And look at the popularity of the (then new) *Physicians' Desk Reference* — it wasn't just physicians who purchased it, he argued, it was laypeople. Yes, the more Art Hayes thought about it, DTC advertising was inevitable.

Then one day, reading the newest issue of *Psychology Today*, everything the new FDA commissioner had been cogitating came together. In an article entitled "Wrongheaded Ideas About Illness," the author Howard Leventhal detailed why more than half of all patients didn't follow doctors' orders about taking prescribed medications. The reason, Leventhal said, was simple: "What patients confronted with illness want is complete and clear information on the threat and on the methods of coping . . . Success or failure in treatment may depend on . . . presenting . . . *an effective image of a coping reaction* [my italics]." Hayes got it: the image was part of the cure! He sat down one day in early February 1982 and, with a staff aide, wrote a speech to be delivered to the staid Pharmaceutical Advertising Council, meeting later that month. Citing Leventhal, Hayes told the group that "it is my impression that [providing an effective image of a coping reaction] is precisely what advertising has been trying to accomplish for over-the-counter drugs for many decades. The question," Hayes asked, "is whether there isn't precisely the same kind of opportunity for communicating effective coping reactions about the proper use of prescription drugs." He believed there was: "we may be on the brink of the exponential growth phase of direct-to-the-consumer promotion of prescription products." To many of the younger ad execs in the room that day, Hayes's speech was nothing short of visionary.

But visions, just like magic, are a transient phenomenon, and things that fire the imagination of the young often go bump in the night for those who have been around a while. Up on Capitol Hill, Hayes's vision quickly warped into the latter. Within a few weeks, he was attacked from every possible quarter, from the administration's natural enemies in Congress to many of his natural allies in academia and at the FDA.

The most damaging charge came in the form of a summons from Representative John Dingell, chairman of the powerful House Subcommittee on Oversight and Investigations. Dingell accused Hayes of misinterpreting the federal code governing prescription drug promotion. Hayes went to the Hill to defend himself. Then came rumblings of dissent from his staff, many of them career bureaucrats who were in no hurry to change the way things had been done for twenty years.

But that was only the beginning of Hayes's troubles. The clincher came in the form of letters to Dingell. The bullheaded congressman hadn't been content with criticizing Hayes; he also sent queries to thirty-six of the nation's leading drug makers, asking them if *they* believed DTC advertising was a good idea and if they *ever* foresaw a time when they might consider undertaking such. All but five responded at length — and in the negative. The biggest names in pharmaceuticals seemed horrified at the very prospect. DTC — direct-to-consumer — was "unprofessional." Things just weren't done that way. Why, it could be "downright dangerous."

In a typical letter, Thomas Collins, chairman of SmithKline French, warned that "advertising would have the objective of driving patients into doctors' offices seeking prescriptions. We believe that the chances for damaging doctor-patient relations and for encouraging costly competitive battles are real, while the likelihood that meaningful patient education will occur is small." The vice president and general counsel of American Home Products, Charles Hagan, put a finer point on it: "DTC advertising would make [patients] extraordinarily susceptible to product promises." The chief of Eli Lilly: "The potential pressures of public advertising of prescription drugs on the scientific decisions of the physician are both unwise and inappropriate." The head of Johnson and Johnson: "[DTC] could adversely affect the traditional patient-physician relationship. Physicians might find themselves having to defend their choice of what they consider an appropriate medication simply because the chosen drug is not heavily advertised and not familiar to the consumer . . . Conversely, a patient may actually demand a particular medication when it might not be the best choice based on the physician's diagnosis or practice."

The handwringing went on and on. At Abbott Laboratories, wrote its chairman, "We believe direct advertising to the consumer introduces a very real possibility of causing harm to patients who may respond to advertisements by pressuring physicians to prescribe medications that may not be required." At Bristol-Myers, said its chief executive, "We fail to understand a benefit to *any* audience" of DTC. Burroughs Wellcome worried that DTC could actually hurt the industry's ability to come up with new drugs because of "the potential for misdirection of industry efforts and resources." The president of Boehringer Ingelheim asked, "Would it be appropriate to push the physician's arm, through the prospective patient-consumer, in his selection of effective therapy? Since the layman cannot be expected to diagnose his or her disease, is it reasonable that he or she be in a position to insist upon a specific treatment?" The senior vice president of Schering-Plough said simply, "We do not believe it is in the public health interest." The president of Searle wrote that it was "dubious that the potential risks could be presented clearly, or, if so, remembered by the consumer." The chiefs of more than a dozen other major firms concurred.

The major medical societies were against DTC as well. Many believed it would lead to widespread self-medication. Worse, "consumers," one physicians' group chief concluded, "will come to regard prescription drugs as any other consumer good." The AMA, according to a congressional staff report prepared later, thought DTC was "fraught with risk of consumer confusion and subversion of the therapeutic relationship between the doctor and patient." The AMA then imposed a ban on DTC in its own patient publications.

With big pharma, Capitol Hill, and his own FDA stacked

against him, Hayes tried to limit the damage and quickly called for a moratorium on the FDA's DTC activities. But to everyone in the official and unofficial world of pharma, it was too late. Arthur Hull Hayes had to go, and in 1983, he did. He had simply gone too far, too quickly.

Or had he? Legally, Hayes was entirely in step with the times. It was perfectly lawful to advertise prescription drugs in 1983, and no one had done more to make that so than Ralph Nader, consumer advocate nonpareil. Among his many projects, Nader had set up the Public Citizen Litigation Group in the early 1970s to take on big consumer-oriented court cases. One of his main concerns was the legal profession, which he regarded as elitist and out of the financial reach of the average consumer. Nader blamed professional collusion: legal societies used state laws to ban the advertising of legal services and fee schedules. Nader saw that as de facto anticompetitive activity that kept the profession insulated from consumer pressure for cheaper services. If you did not know that some lawyers worked for cheaper rates than others, how could you exercise your market power as an individual?

To find the right case, Nader hired a young New York attorney named Alan Morrison. The son of socially concerned parents, Morrison was a natural Naderite; he had read Nader's books and was drawn, he later recalled, to the great "battle over corporate dominance." The ban on legal advertising was just one more way that the system kept legal services from the poor.

But try as he might, Morrison could not find the right case for Nader's legal advertising battle. Yes, there were a lot of upstart lawyers who might serve as plaintiffs, but he wasn't likely to curry a lot of public support or jurisprudential sympathy for a case that looked as if it would benefit only attorneys. "I realized that such a case would be more sympathetic if litigated from the customer side. The first case should not be *for* lawyers." He waited. Then, in 1976, a strange little court action crossed his desk. It had been referred by a small nonprofit organization, the Virginia Citizens Consumer Council. The council had taken on the state of Virginia's Board of Pharmacy for its rules forbidding advertising of prescription drug prices by retail pharmacists.

Like similar laws in many other states, the pharmacy board had long held that advertising of prescription drugs would cause too much competition, resulting in the degradation of pharmacy professionalism and, eventually, the destruction of the pharmacist-customer relationship. In essence, people would lose respect for the profession if it advertised. It was the same case that legal and medical societies, from the ABA to the AMA, often made when defending their bans on advertising. Yet at its heart was an unyielding and, for the times, indigestible assumption: people had to be protected from information because they would inevitably use the information in a stupid, ignorant, and ultimately self-destructive way. That reasoning struck the Virginia Citizens Consumer Council as fundamentally patronizing and antidemocratic, particularly when one looked at an important fact: the poor were the most likely to suffer from not knowing which pharmacy sold drugs for the best price. The council sued the Board of Pharmacy and won at the district court level, and now it fell to Morrison to defend the victory when the board appealed it to the Supreme Court in 1976.

The core of the federal case, as advanced by the pharmacy board, focused on the issue of commercial speech. Using an older doctrine which held that commercial speech was not protected by the First Amendment, the board argued that the state was well within its constitutional powers to restrict what pharmacists could say. But Morrison was a crafty court watcher, and he intuited that the Court would be disinclined to buy an argument based on traditional free speech law. Increasingly, first in a 1972 case known as *Kleindienst v. Mandel*, then in a 1985 case known as *Bigelow*, the Court majority had articulated a new doctrine called "the hearer's right to know." In other words, it was not just the speaker who was protected by the First Amendment, it was also the potential hearer of information. Morrison boiled all of this down to one compelling case. "The hearer has rights! And rights to hear an advertisement that was factual! That was my case. It all boiled down to access to safe, lawful medical services, and in my case it was access to information about safe prescription drugs." The Court agreed, and in a seven-to-one decision, again found in favor of the Citizens Consumer Council.

But in doing so, Justice Harry Blackmun extended the protection of commercial speech beyond what anyone — Morrison included — had anticipated. In *Bigelow* and *Kleindienst*, part of the reason advertisements were held protectable — the government could not enact laws to restrict them — was that in those cases the ads had conveyed something deemed socially or politically relevant, something of a higher purpose than a mere commercial transaction. By contrast, in the *Virginia Pharmacy* case, the only "speech" at issue was, as Justice Blackmun put it, the ability of the pharmacist to say "I will sell you X prescription drug at Y price." Should such purely commercial speech lack all First Amendment protection? Blackmun and the majority said it did not. "As to the particular consumer's interest in the free flow of commercial information, that interest may be keener, if not keener by far, than the interest in the day's most urgent political debate," Blackmun wrote. "Those whom the suppression of prescription drug price information hits the hardest are the poor, the sick, and particularly the aged. A disproportionate amount of their income tends to be spent on prescription drugs; yet they are the least able to learn, by shopping from pharmacist to pharmacist, where their scarce dollars are best spent." Blackmun had created the "consumer's right to know."

And that right to know, or right to hear, extended to society in general, said Blackmun. "Advertising, however tasteless and excessive it may seem, is nonetheless dissemination of information as to who is producing and selling what product, for what reason, and at what price. So long as we preserve a predominantly free enterprise economy, the allocation of our resources in large measure will be made through numerous private economic decisions. It is a matter of public interest that those decisions, in the aggregate, be intelligent and well informed. To this end, the free flow of information is indispensable."

Couched in the growing social and consumer issues of the day, Blackmun's soliloquy hit home; it was, in a sense, part and parcel of a growing notion, sometimes heard in liberal circles, sometimes heard in conservative ones, that by freeing industry from its old boundaries on disseminating information, one could empower consumers. It was a potent, deeply American idea with optimism at its core, a primal enunciation of the proverbial win-win doctrine of social change that now inflects just about any serious policy discussion in this country. Change that benefits all and hurts none — who could argue with that?

There was a dissenter in the Virginia case, and he was no lightweight. William Rehnquist was the Court's most conservative justice, and he was unswayed by the happy talk. As far as he was concerned, the First Amendment was an instrument to protect public decision making in a democracy — period. "I had understood this view to relate to . . . political, social, and other public issues, rather than the decision of a particular individual as to whether to purchase one or another kind of shampoo," Rehnquist wrote. Worse, he argued, where would industry take this new freedom? Might we next see advertisements that said things like "Pain getting you down? Insist that your physician prescribe Demerol," the future chief justice jabbed. "You pay a little more than for aspirin, but you get a lot more relief." He went on, clearly having some fun: "Don't spend another sleepless night. Ask your doctor about Seconal without delay." No, no, no! said a now very serious Rehnquist. "The societal interest against the promotion of drug use for every ill, real or imaginary, seems to me extremely strong."

But *Virginia* was now the law of the land. And in the advertising industry of the eighties, young, often idealistic men and women were looking for ways to exploit it as Blackmun, Morrison, and Nader could never have imagined.

In 1981, Joe Davis was a senior advertising executive at the esteemed Ogilvy Agency in New York, overseeing a broad line of over-the-counter drug ads for Bristol-Myers and Ciba-Geigy. Davis had always been a bookish fellow, inclined toward tomes that, as he put it, "stretched my mind." One recently published polemic, *Medical Nemesis*, blew his mind. *Nemesis* was not exactly a *New York Times* bestseller, but its author, a former Catholic priest named Ivan Illich, managed to get his ideas out to a lot of influential people. He was a product of the times. An iconoclast par excellence, Illich had made a name for himself by writing a series of books, one on education, one on transportation, and now one on institutional medicine, which detailed brilliantly how the institutions of modern life had become counterproductive: School systems had become so hierarchical and bureaucratic that true learning had become virtually impossible. (Illich went so far as to say we should get rid of them.) Likewise, departments of transportation had become so fixated on the creation of highways that human beings found themselves unable to get around unless they had cars. (The solution was to get rid of highways.) And medicine, Illich said, had become so profit-driven, diagnostic, and scientific as to become "a major threat to health." Doctors caused more pain than relief. To a generation of young medical men and women, Illich struck a chord; certainly he was part of the background music to activist physicians like Terry Kupers and his band of antipharma interns, and he was likely one of the cultural critics of big pharma who had made Donald Rumsfeld, during his days at G. D. Searle, so glum. Illich's work, particularly one passage, hit home with Joe Davis: "Before sickness came to be perceived primarily as an organic or behavioral abnormality," Illich wrote,

> he who got sick could still find in the eyes of the doctor a reflection of his own anguish and some recognition of the uniqueness of his suffering. Now, what he meets is the gaze of a biological accountant engaged in input/output calculations. His sickness is taken from him and turned into the raw material for an institutional enterprise. His condition is interpreted according to a set of abstract rules in a language he cannot understand. He is taught about alien entities that the doctor combats, but only just as much as the doctor considers necessary to gain the patient's cooperation. Language is taken over by the doctors: the sick person is deprived of meaningful words for his anguish, which is thus further increased by linguistic mystification.

It was a powerful point. As Davis recalls, "It was one of those books that could change people's lives, and I recall sitting there and underlining whole passages." He began discussing the ideas with friends in the ad industry. "Pretty soon I began to think of putting Ivan Illich's ideas into the pharma advertising world as a way of getting people more engaged in their own symptomology and care." Of course, it was Illich's analysis — that people had become distanced from understanding their own bodies — and not his cure — that they should avoid the medical establishment like the plague — that registered with Davis. Advertising, he came to believe, could reintegrate people into their own health care. Where Arthur Hull Hayes saw the therapeutic value of a "coping image," Joe Davis intuited the empowering role of the written and spoken word.

There were other forward-thinking people in medical advertising, too. A friend of Davis's, William Castagnoli, had been chafing for years to try out direct-to-consumer advertising, but had made little headway. Castagnoli had made his bones at the old Frohlich Pharmaceutical Advertising Agency, which, under its founder, Arthur Frohlich, became a veritable monopoly for medical journal advertising. In the mid-1980s, at Medicus, the successor agency after Frohlich died, Castagnoli served as a senior executive overlooking the Merrill-Dow account. He had tried to get his superiors interested in DTC for prescription drugs. Unfortunately for him, the industry — as evidenced in the backpedaling over poor old Arthur Hull Hayes — was in no rush to repeat that debacle. Still, Castagnoli paid attention to small things happening in the field, and, like Hayes, he believed that DTC was not only the right thing, it was also inevitable. A British company, Boots Pharmaceuticals, had proved that to him when, out of nowhere and without consulting the traditional pharma-FDA-advertising axis, they began advertising a new prescription painkiller, Rufen. The FDA eventually came down on the firm, but Boots sold a ton of Rufen in the process. Everyone in the industry was talking about it, albeit in the disdainful way that so irked Bill Castagnoli. "They pissed all over it."

In 1985, Castagnoli was put in charge of the launch of a new drug for Merrill, an antihistamine called Seldane. Merrill had spent lots of money developing the drug, even more getting it approved by the FDA. It had done so because it believed Seldane was a huge advance over previous generations of antihistamines:

the drug did not make people drowsy. Yet as Castagnoli and Davis, now working together, looked at the market analysis of the drug, all they saw were problems. The biggest was that people with allergies rarely visited their doctors unless they were very sick; the average length between visits was three years. If they had problems, they often simply switched, on their own, to other existing over-the-counter medications. "If we relied on the traditional way of doing things, using medical journal ads directed at physicians, you would have to wait three years for this trickle-down to start resulting in sales," Davis recalls. The obvious solution was to somehow "drive patients to their doctors." But in 1984 the FDA had imposed a moratorium on DTC. And while advertising drug prices was legal, advertising specific drugs and their specific therapeutic benefits was a tricky matter, with the FDA exercising special regulatory powers that required lengthy, often off-putting safety information that would make the ads both ineffective and, especially on TV, expensive.

Then the pair had a brainstorm. What if they advertised *not* the therapeutic effect of Seldane — that it helped you get unclogged — but instead that "a new drug for allergies is out" and that "it does not make you drowsy"? If a patient wanted to find out more, "Go and see your doctor." And by not naming the drug, the ad could hint at obvious benefits: if you were not drowsy at work, you could do your job better. In fact, forget the whole notion of hyping a cure — go for the feeling, go for the career! Jerry Weinstein, Castagnoli's creative director, came up with a brilliant tagline for the campaign: "Now you can put your hay fever to sleep while you stay awake!" And work, work, work!

The troika then launched a campaign to reeducate the media itself. At *Time* magazine, "they knew everything about whiskey and cars but nothing about health care," Davis recalls. He and Castagnoli tutored the magazine about arcane FDA rules, the definition of "over-the-counter" versus "prescription," what constituted a promotion, and so on. They did the same act for the *New York Times* Sunday supplement group. At CBS, still stinging from the Hayes incident, lawyers were less than enthusiastic. Davis and Weinstein showed them a proposed commercial. All it said was that there was a new kind of medication for allergy sufferers that did not make you drowsy. It then showed a young, attractive nurse coming out to meet a patient and saying, "The doctor will see you now." Weinstein recalls that the next day, he got a jubilant phone call from CBS executives. "They were so excited," he recalls. "Once they thought about the implications, they knew there was a huge and fresh flow of new money there."

The Seldane campaign, launched in 1988, became one of Medicus's, and Merrill's, most successful campaigns ever. Sales of Seldane soared beyond anyone's wildest imaginations. Merrill could not manufacture it fast enough. This result was all the more remarkable, given the low-key approach of Weinstein's copy. As Castagnoli says: "We were idealistic. We wanted it to be almost journalistic. Almost a public service. Here are the facts. Your doctor is the one who can explain it to you. Period. No emotion. No product name."

But no emotion — and especially no product name — was not exactly a rallying cry to others in the advertising industry, particularly those on the big-dollar TV side, who had just had their appetites whetted. Pharmaceutical CEOs could get only so excited about quasi-public service, they said, and they would part with only so much money for DTC. To really bring them around, you would first have to get rid of the FDA's opposition to DTC, and to do that, you would first have to soften up the AMA, which set the tone on such things.

The opportunity to do that came about just as serendipitously as Joe Davis reading Ivan Illich.

In 1989, the head of the pharmaceutical giant Upjohn, Dr. Theodore Cooper, had a problem. A distinguished cardiologist, public health advocate, and researcher, Cooper was used to dealing with troublesome, complex issues. He had initiated the high blood pressure project of the NIH in the 1970s, when many in medicine and government were not exactly comfortable with the idea of governmental meddling in chronic disease management. The project became a model for scores of other major public health initiatives. But the discontent percolating at Upjohn, to which he had come fairly late in his career, was totally foreign to Cooper: Men were not buying the company's new antibalding medication, Rogaine. The reason for that was a classic. When physicians prescribed it, they simply parroted the boilerplate instructions provided by Upjohn: apply the cream first thing in the morning. Men, who have been known by some to be somewhat literal-minded, had done just that — and then promptly took their morning shower, in the process diluting the Rogaine. The result was that Rogaine did not work, and men were not renewing their prescriptions, a potential billion-dollar bust. Somehow, Upjohn had to get the message out fast to physicians about how to prescribe the drug properly.

So Cooper called an old college friend, Jim Sammons, the executive vice president of the American Medical Association. Sammons, a charming southerner, was no medical visionary, but rather a financial innovator. In just a few years he had transformed the AMA, which had fallen on hard times, into an economic powerhouse, or, as he put it, "a modern corporation." Sammons was sympathetic to Cooper's woes, and, with his new vice president of marketing, Wendy Borow-Johnson, flew down to Upjohn's Kalamazoo headquarters for a meeting. As the two men talked, Borow-Johnson realized that many of the same problems that so frustrated Ted Cooper — mainly the inability to talk directly and accurately to patients — also confronted many members of the AMA. For them the issue was managed care, the new beast on the medical scene, which, through its intrusive ways of rationing care, often made patients very resentful. Under Wendy Borow-Johnson, the AMA marketing department had responded by producing a series of profession-burnishing trailers, aired in movie theaters, called "First Comes Caring." Traveling back to Chicago with Sammons and contemplating Cooper's woes, then trying to reconcile them with the AMA's ban on DTC, she "pointed out how inconsistent it was that we could be doing all these things to promote patient information and proactive patient-physician relationships and then say essentially, 'No, patients can't handle information about drugs.'" The pair went back and created a new informational ad aimed at physicians called "How to Talk to Your Patient." It was a big hit.

And why not DTC drug ads? Borow-Johnson argued. "Times have changed," she recalls telling her boss. "Why would you limit the ability to give information to patients? When my mother had me, she had only Dr. Spock. When I had my baby I had a hundred videos and books. Why wouldn't you allow this?"

Richard Corlin, then the vice speaker of the AMA, was convinced that DTC was now a *fait accompli* — "the train was leaving the station," he later recalled — and he commissioned an AMA committee to look into the matter of ending the association's 1984 blanket ban on DTC ads. In 1992, that committee commenced a series of discussions, which were attended by both FDA staffers and a number of pharmaceutical executives. (The AMA would not release the names of the latter.) By mid-1992, the committee made a formal recommendation to the AMA General Assembly to rescind the old ban. Only one delegate spoke out against it. The AMA had voted to push the physician's arm.

The courts, the advertising industry, big pharma, and the AMA: by 1995, almost everyone was coming around to the great possibilities of marrying prescription drugs with the modern media. Everyone, that is, except David Kessler and his FDA. Kessler, who had eagerly embraced Gerry Mossinghoff's idea for user fees, was turning out to be a nightmare for pharma's media dreams. He didn't like the idea of DTC at all. DTC, he said, would distort and interrupt the proper functioning of the doctor-patient relationship. Worse were Kessler's views on the subject of medical marketing. He hated a growing practice by drug makers and their marketing representatives known as off-label promotion.

"Off-label promotion" is the term used for a pharmaceutical company's advocacy of a prescription drug for a use that the FDA has not specifically approved. Often, this type of advertising involves the distribution of medical journal articles that discuss such uses — Paxil for shyness, for example — with the intent of subtly encouraging physicians to, let's just say it, experiment. Off-label prescribing, particularly in the last-ditch treatment of acute diseases, like cancer, can often hold tremendous promise, but when it comes to chronic diseases, it often causes more pain than relief. Such was the case, in 1989, with the drug Tambocor, officially indicated for major arrhythmia but overprescribed for years for minor arrhythmia, causing, by several counts, more than 50,000 deaths. Of course, it is entirely legal for a physician to prescribe a drug for any reason he or she deems fit, but there has always been a thin line between what a drug company might do to educate about such uses and what a drug company might do to promote such uses. Until Kessler, the FDA had adopted a laissez-faire attitude except in the most egregious cases of hard sell.

But Kessler was convinced by what he perceived as a growing brazenness by drug firms to promote their products in illegal, or at least supralegal, ways. He was not entirely off base. Ever since the reality of generic competition began to hit home in pharma executive suites, the hard sell had become a way of life for pharma sales reps. At the FDA's Division of Drug Marketing, Advertising, and Communications (DDMAC), a small and traditionally underfunded unit dedicated to making sure that drug ads to physicians were accurate and balanced, evidence of the trend was clear. On September 6, 1994, for example, DDMAC obtained compelling evidence that sales representatives of SmithKline, makers of Paxil, were handing out unapproved, homemade promotional materials containing false and misleading claims. One of the items was a handwritten note, on Paxil stationery, left with physicians. "Dr. [X]. Hello!," it said. "Why should you use Paxil instead of Prozac?" It then went on to suggest that Paxil was safer than Prozac (it is not), that it cost less (only to wholesalers), and that it was easier on the elderly (a claim that was, by any stretch of the scientific imagination, utterly false).

Pfizer was no better. On August 12, 1994, DDMAC amassed evidence that the firm was hyping its new antidepressant Zoloft beyond the limits of any known research. The agency ordered

Pfizer to discontinue a whole raft of promotional materials, because, among other things, the items "minimized adverse event data," downplayed the risk of toxicity, made bloated claims of "broad spectrum efficacy," and used bogus rates of side-effect reporting.

Prozac maker Eli Lilly took things one step further by sponsoring a National Depression Awareness Day at a Maryland high school, giving out promotional pens and brochures — a perk once limited to physicians who actually knew something about the disease — to 1,300 students.

By late 1994, Kessler was so angered by the trend that he sent one of his deputy commissioners to testify before the House Subcommittee on Regulation, Business Opportunities, and Technology, stating that "promotion of unapproved uses by company sales representatives is a major problem." Kessler then decided to redeploy the DDMAC to go after the culprits. To many members of the medical marketing and ad community, Dr. Kessler had declared war.

All of this seemed somewhat strange to John Kamp, then the new senior vice president of the powerful American Association of Advertising Agencies, or AAAA. He was puzzled when members of the AAAA, some of the most aggressive advertising agencies in the world, came complaining about Kessler. "I asked them, 'Didn't the FDA believe in the First Amendment?'" he recalls. The advertisers' response was one of fear: they did not want a recap of the Dingell inquisition of 1983; they did not want to get hauled up in front of Congress only to find the pharma CEOs getting soft again. Finally, Kamp got four of the AAAA's most powerful members — executives from what is now Grey Advertising among them — to let him undertake an aggressive "reeducation" campaign of David Kessler's FDA. Why? "Because it was an important advertising category that they couldn't get."

Says Kamp, "We intentionally got on the speakers circuit where DDMAC people would be and we showed them very openly what we were concerned with. We had to get them to see that advertising was a form of consumer information — we had to get them to see themselves as regulators of consumer information." He also chipped away at Kessler's inconsistencies in logic. How could someone so fervently against smoking be so opposed to DTC ads for something as innocuous, safe, but potentially lifesaving, as the nicotine patch?

Yet anyone who has ever tried to change anything about the FDA knows one thing: it does not necessarily respond to reason. It responds to threat. So Kamp and the AAAA began pumping money into the Washington Legal Foundation (WLF), a conservative legal advocacy group with a wide and deep network of like-minded attorneys willing to take on just about any government agency that impeded free enterprise. The driving force behind the WLF was a man named Dan Popeo, and, as it happened, Dan Popeo had a personal bone to pick with the FDA. Five close friends of his had died of cancer in recent years; one was the close friend of his young son. Witnessing that tragedy, Popeo saw first-hand how FDA limits on off-label information had impeded the care of the boy. As Popeo saw it, "government was practicing medicine — it had gone way beyond safety and efficacy, and that was troubling to me." In 1994, he had the WLF file a court action against Kessler and the FDA for suppressing patient, physician, and industry First Amendment rights. In 1995, the WLF also filed a citizen petition calling on the FDA to relax its regulations, citing "procedures [that] are inherently chilling and inconsistent with the First Amendment because they constitute a prior restraint on free speech." As Kamp recalls, "That got Kessler's attention."

By joining with the WLF, Kamp got access to a growing cadre of conservative legal scholars. One of them, Dan Troy, also worked for the AAAA's law firm, Wiley Rein and Fielding, and that was an enormous advantage as well. The firm was legendary for its ecumenism, comfortable with commercial clients like the AAAA and all the major TV networks (limousine-liberal and otherwise), as well as civil libertarians and various public inter-est groups. Dan Troy was a natural for the assault. He had clerked for Robert Bork and had already defended tobacco companies against Kessler's attempts to curtail their advertising. Troy was also a legal scholar of sorts, published in both academic and popular conservative magazines and newspapers, and a fellow at the conservative American Enterprise Institute. He was a long-standing member of the Federalist Society, an organization of conservative and libertarian attorneys who — via a close reading of the Founding Fathers — favored strict limits on federal regulation of industry. Among liberals, of course, Troy was vilified. Among conservatives, Troy was a new star, unintimidated by prevailing D.C. sentiment and willing to take on powerful institutions of government that inhibited free enterprise and impinged on commercial — and by extension private — liberties. He was, by almost every measure, a true believer, channeling the Founding Fathers in brilliant ways that would, he hoped, make everyone else one as well.

Troy's most important assignment, at least as far as Kamp and his Madison Avenue clients were concerned, was clear. He needed to continue to erode the distinction between public and commercial speech, in the process whittling away at the FDA's anti-DTC inclinations and off-label hostility. This Troy did in a memorable friend-of-the-court brief in a case known as *44 Liquormart v. Rhode Island*, in which the issue was the state's authority to prohibit liquor price advertising at places other than the point of purchase. Arguing a strict constructionist theory in front of an increasingly conservative, strict constructionist court, Troy focused on the intentions of the Founders when it came to the First Amendment and advertising. Examining a range of eighteenth-century newspapers and their publishers, including Benjamin Franklin, Troy told the court that "Colonial Americans plainly viewed the freedom of speech as protecting far more than just political speech." He did not dwell on one countervailing fact: That this lack of distinction between commercial and public speech was likely because most Colonial newspapers were *primarily* vehicles for advertising, hardly the impartial beacons that modern papers are expected to be. Instead, Troy told the court, "There is no evidence on the other side — nothing at all — to suggest that, as an original matter, commercial messages should be treated differently from other types of messages."

As Troy talked, so did the justices listen. The court was unanimous in striking down the Rhode Island law. He had particularly won over some of the newer members. Justice Clarence Thomas relied on the Troy doctrine in rejecting any "philosophical or historical basis for asserting that commercial speech is of 'lower value' than 'noncommercial speech.'" Antonin Scalia was moved to riff that he shared the majority's "aversion toward paternalistic governmental policies that prevent men and women from hearing facts that might not be good for them." Troy had prevailed.

Whether one agreed with the rhetoric, at the FDA, minds have been known to change when courts begin to riff. "The cases were starting to focus their minds," Kamp says. "They were concerned that they were vulnerable." One consequence of that new "focus" was a new willingness to consider DTC advertising and, the Holy Grail of Madison Avenue, rescinding the costly "brief summary" requirement. Madison Avenue hated the summary because it was anything but brief, often running on for minutes at a time with an emotionally deadening list of side effects, cautions, hedging ifs, ands, and buts. So, in a 1995 FDA hearing, Kamp orchestrated a series of testimonies about the importance of DTC, and how it was only possible to do DTC if the FDA rescinded the brief summary requirement — or at least made it very, very brief.

Now even big pharma was willing to make its case. The most stunning turnaround came from American Home Products, which had argued so indignantly in 1984 that "DTC advertising would make [patients] extraordinarily susceptible to product promises." Nancy Buc, a former FDA counsel turned American Home attorney, turned the argument upside down: "Empowering the patient as well as the physician with information increases the likelihood that someone — patient, friend or relative of the patient, or physician — will get the dialogue started. Getting the dialogue started is key to avoiding underuse as well as overuse of prescription drugs, to proper weighing of risk factors, to consumers' understanding why and when and how to take the drugs, the whole process of intelligent and careful and proper prescribing."

And the key to doing that, witness after witness testified, was to get rid of the brief summary requirement. Not only did the rule make TV ads too costly, necessitating a long rollout of detailed safety and fair-balance information, but it also made the ads ineffective and even hurtful. In other words, too much information was bad! As Jon Schommer, a professor from Ohio State who had done research for a pharma trade group, amazingly testified: "The ad might trigger [an] information search, and [patients] might actually read that blasted brief summary, because 'It is my health, I am on the drug, I am going to try to tackle this information because I want to learn more about my drug.' And if that person would start reading the brief summary of information, they might become overloaded . . . 'I can't understand all this technical talk. I am completely overloaded. I give up. I am going to stop taking my medication.'" The underlying logic was thus: Expensive, lengthy information, bad. Cheap, short information, good.

The whole thing was a bit much for Irv Lerner, the former head of Roche. "I thought it was a huge mistake then and I think the same now. It whittles down the power of the physician and, frankly, it hurts the image of the industry by lining pharma up with beer and tobacco and cosmetics."

But such concerns were largely brushed aside by the FDA committee hearing the witnesses. The objectors all sounded like the kind of folk that Justices Scalia and Thomas disliked so much, what with all their paternalistic governmental policies. By the end of the hearings, a consensus had clearly formed. As Bob Temple, then the powerful head of the FDA's drug evaluation division, said to John Kamp not long after: "The brief summary is going to go the way of the Holy Roman Empire." By 1997, the agency had rolled back the requirement, clearing the way for an avalanche of new pharma TV ads. It was party time among the broadcast clients at Wiley Rein.

The party shifted into higher gear in 1999, when a district court judge finally ruled on the original off-label case, to the favor of the Washington Legal Foundation (and, by monetary daisy chain, Wiley, the AAAA, and medical marketers). Again, the key to the win was the antipaternalism argument. The government "cannot justify a restriction of truthful, non-misleading speech on the paternalistic assumption that such restriction is necessary to protect the listener from ignorantly or inadvertently misusing the information," the court wrote.

Of course, that "non-misleading" part — that could be tricky. Should a drug company be able to distribute, via highly trained and restrained medical affairs people, studies showing that a drug for one approved purpose also "seemed" to help kids, with, say, stage-four brain cancer, an unapproved use? The average fellow would likely say yes. But should a drug company also be allowed, as has been the case with antidepressants, to dispatch tens of thousands of young, barely trained sales reps, most just out of college, to hand out to general practitioners, with no experience in psychiatry, studies that "suggest" that adult antidepressants "might" help kids with depressions? The murk blossoms anew. The FDA's traditional response was to come down hard on the latter cases, and it intended to protect its powers to do so by appealing the court decision.

But again the FDA lost. The case was upheld in 2002, with Wiley Rein itself at the helm. By then there was, apparently, too much to lose to let some conservative think tank handle it. Now the legal right of pills to speak had become a very mainstream notion. The "consumer's right to know" — Ralph Nader and Alan Morrison's great triumph of the 1970s — had become the corporation's right to "subtly encourage." Put another way, the reigning governmental, legal, and political ethos about prescription drug promotion had morphed from "patient trust thy doctor" into "buyer beware."

The immediate result was an explosion of economic activity — the creation of two new information industries, one based on DTC, one based on off-label promotion. The former was the sexier. By 2003 big pharma was spending upwards of $3 billion a year on DTC, almost all of it, it might be noted, on drugs for chronic diseases and not on acute conditions like childhood cancer. Pfizer alone spent more than half a billion. DTC became the province of Madison Avenue's most powerful ad agencies and, of course, their Wiley Rein broadcaster clients — the publicly licensed theater of the new DTC world — sans, of course, any troublingly patronizing brief summaries that might confuse the poor patient.

With the money came the so-called creative influence. DTC was no longer just about giving patients useful information. Soon there were commercials for Paxil for social anxiety disorder, promising to "help you become yourself again." Talent agencies began packaging celebrities with pills. The tennis star Monica Seles, apparently employing a long-hidden expertise in brain chemistry, became the spokeswoman for prescription migraine pills. Lynda Carter, once known for portraying Wonder Woman, now deployed her superpowers to talk up drugs for irritable bowel syndrome. Ads for Viagra showed fat, balding men partying in the street. Celebrex spots showed arthritics dancing in the street. There were ads for GERD and ads for toenail fungus relief. There were ads for Claritin that had no information at all — just pretty people running through pretty fields of flowers. And on the Web, where DTC was flourishing, the ethos morphed again. As the trade magazine *Medical Marketing and Media* stated, the "three principles of a good pharmaceutical-brand Web site" were: "Be the brand." "Don't forget the audience." "Always persuade."

Many of the new ads left some older ad people, particularly folks like Bill Castagnoli and Joe Davis, feeling a bit betrayed. "It was all supposed to be about getting a person to the doctor," Castagnoli says, "not an emotional thing that just raised expectations. It broke our hearts."

Off-label marketing grew even more quickly. By 2000 there were dozens of pharmaceutical marketing congresses springing up all over the country, making the world safe from paternalism. Their overall mission was to find ways to use the new information industries — data mining, the Internet — to convince doctors to try drugs for promising, if unproved, uses. Increasingly, drug marketers saw physicians as sales partners, whom they treated to elaborate "conventions" in such scientific citadels as Las Vegas, Miami Beach, and New Orleans. One good indicator of their success: Neurontin, an older drug indicated for epilepsy, was now one of pharma's biggest billion-dollar babies. The reason: almost 80 percent of its sales came from off-label uses, everything from bipolar disorder to chronic pain to attention deficit disorder.

And, more and more, the writing of a prescription served an entirely different purpose from that of simply delivering a potentially helpful molecule into a patient's bloodstream. Just like DTC, with its many balletic arthritics, the prescription, with its official-looking spareness and illegible Latin scrawl, became part of medical theater. And that theater had an economic function. It signaled the end of a short, managed-care doctor's visit with a tangible sign of treatment. A salesman might call it "the closer." Arthur Hull Hayes might have called it the "coping image."

And what of Arthur Hull Hayes? Like many who had helped pills learn to talk, he had made a soft landing, first as an executive at a pharmaceuticals company and then at Nelson Communications, one of the biggest health care advertising agencies in the nation and a subsidiary of Publicis Healthcare Group, the biggest DTC and off-label marketing firm in the world.

And what of Dan Troy? In February 2002, he was made general counsel of the Food and Drug Administration. At about the same time, warning letters to drug companies for deceptive ads — traditionally the leading indicator of FDA vigilance — dropped by two thirds. Even the pharmaceuticals trade press was stunned by the change, noting, in one headline, that now "most medical promotion is out of sight of regulators."

Quietly that same year, Seldane, the drug that launched the DTC revolution, was pulled from the market. It caused heart problems.

BIG PHARMA REBORN: HOW PHARMACEUTICAL EXECUTIVES MADE THEIR COMPANIES EVERYBODY'S BEST FRIEND

With the regulatory, legal, and media playing fields retooled in their favor, big pharma CEOs began turning to what, deep in their hearts, they knew was the real problem: the management of the very companies they commanded. On the eve of the generic competition about to be unleashed by the Hatch-Waxman bill, almost every pharma company still followed the old, postwar business model. Departments were highly structured and distinct. Scientists did not talk to marketing people, who did not talk to finance people, who did not talk to regulatory people, who did not talk to legal people. "The mindset was very patent-leather shoe, very country club," a PMA executive observed. It was a mindset slow to innovate and hesitant to establish new precedents.

The experience of the typical pharma leaders was thus increasingly summed up in two words: status anxiety. Whereas in the past they had floated along on the safe raft of patent protection, content to pop out a new drug every few years, now they sailed a ship of multiple incipient leaks. Their boards of directors, also frightened of patent expiration, pushed for more, faster, and all in a leaner, cost-conscious fashion. Those same boards — made up of everyone from the heads of American Express and AT&T to former senators and government regulators — were also pressing pharma CEOs to understand something else: they had to start heeding a new master, the personal investor. New forces in the economy — principally mutual funds and the emerging consumer financial industry, in turn driven by people who read publications like *Money* and *Personal Investor* — were no longer happy with 10, 11, or even 12 percent annual returns. Given the cost of their stock, they wanted 14, 15, 16 — even 20 percent! Men like Roche CEO Irv Lerner, long treated as semi-royalty within their own preserves, now faced the classic entrepreneurial dilemma: innovate or die.

In response, Lerner conjured a "guidance" policy that, while meant to cure Roche, was adaptable to the entire industry. "As I saw it, we had to do four things, and we had to do them very well and very fast. First, we had to make the most of what we had already," Lerner said. "Second, we had to make our research and development department be much more productive. Third, we had to supplement what we had with alliances with other companies. And then, fourth, we had to strategically acquire new drugs from outside the company." Almost immediately after the passage of Hatch-Waxman, nearly every other pharma CEO launched a similar quest. Notably, almost all of them focused exclusively on drugs for chronic disease, from cardiovascular and gastrointestinal illnesses to depression to diabetes. The response was so uniform that the many in both business and the academy would eventually describe it as "the end of infectious disease."

It was also the beginning of a new pharmaceutical era. To wit: of the four missions articulated by Lerner, the first — making the most of what one had — would be brilliantly launched not by a traditional country-club American, schooled in the ways of Harvard or Yale, but rather, by a young Dane who, only a decade earlier, had been a world-class tennis star.

Jan Leschly, in 1979 the new head of the pharmaceuticals division of Squibb, was fond of practicing his backhand and forehand — even when he wasn't playing tennis. Tall, handsome, preternaturally tanned and charming, Leschly was a fierce competitor, so fierce that many of his own pharma colleagues, both in and out of Squibb, often wished he were still playing tennis instead of making their lives so uncomfortable. "If you're not keeping score, you're just practicing!" he liked to exhort his executives. Or "I never stepped on the court without expecting to win!" And that was Leschly at breakfast.

Leschly came to Squibb, a 125-year-old conglomerate of candy, vitamins, drugs and toothbrushes, via an unusual route. The son of a Danish brewer, he went to college in the late 1950s, majoring in business and pharmacy, intending to follow in his father's footsteps. Instead, he entered the professional tennis world, where he played alongside Ilie Nastasi and Jörgen Ulrich, two of the era's greats. For a decade, Leschly bombed around the European tennis circuit, eventually coming under the sponsorship of Novo, a Danish pharmaceuticals company. By the early 1980s, he attracted the interest of Novo's chief executive, who groomed him for a job in the marketing department. Eventually Leschly took up the offer. He proved a fast study, and by the late 1970s, he had transformed the marketing of insulin at Novo.

Unfortunately, Leschly's hard-driving ways — and his pushi-
ness at development meetings to focus almost exclusively on
drugs that had huge market potential — eventually alienated
him from his mentor, a more traditional medical man with an inclination toward scientific breakthroughs. The Leschly career
train stopped.

But only momentarily. In 1979, Leschly got a call from Richard
Furlaud, Squibb's chief executive. Furlaud was a quietly patient
man who, for almost fifteen years, had been trying to transform
Squibb from an also-ran conglomerate into a profitable "drug
house," as they were then known. Furlaud knew part of the problem: Squibb was just too traditional, too old-school. Nobody
talked to each other. "Nobody danced with the other guys' wives
at company parties!" The company needed a jolt of charm and
energy, and Leschly appeared straight out of central casting.

As one of Leschly's first tests, Furlaud proffered a drug, just
nearing FDA approval, that was fraught with both opportunity
and peril. The drug, Capoten, was indicated for treatment of high
blood pressure, and it was a breakthrough, the first in a new class
of drugs for a condition that affected millions. Capoten was what
we now know as an ACE inhibitor, working on the complex system of enzymes that govern vascular constriction. It seemed to
work without many of the side effects of diuretics, the usual
treatment. Furlaud had spent a bundle on Capoten, and his board
was excited about it. Wall Street analysts were predicting a $2
billion market. This was the drug that would remake Squibb.

But try as Furlaud might, by 1984 Capoten was still struggling
for market share due to reports of side effects in clinical trials in
Japan. When the FDA finally got around to approving Capoten, it
was for only a small market of "last measures" treatment — for
people with one foot in the grave. Almost immediately new science emerged suggesting that the side effects were not so bad
as feared, and that they could be eliminated by decreasing the
drug's dosage. Capoten got the broad application approval in
1984, but Capoten sales stayed in the doldrums, a situation made
worse by the fact that Merck, in 1985, won approval for a similar
drug to be marketed as a first-line treatment. It was, for all in-
tents and purposes, identical to Capoten, but doctors were in-

clined to prescribe it because it had not come smudged with (as it turned out unwarranted) safety warnings.

As Leschly saw it, the problem was all about perception. Squibb had allowed others to control the medical-media environment instead of being proactive. His first move was to reinvigorate the sales corps, hiring five hundred new employees to detail the drug nationwide; he made it a point to travel to regional sales offices, something no other Squibb executive had done. Then there was the issue of the side effects. To deal with that, Leschly mined the Squibb research department, which had been looking at the chemical sulfhydryl, the component of Capoten first suspected of causing lowered white blood cell counts in Japan. Researchers had found something else unsuspected about the drug: it seemed to help contain some of the deterioration that occurred after a heart attack. The data were preliminary, but Leschly armed his sales force with it and used it to push back against Merck. Sales improved.

Then Leschly did something utterly unprecedented. Through the Squibb Foundation, he underwrote an extensive study of the quality of life of patients who were on different forms of hypertensive drug therapy. This tack was fundamentally different. Instead of focusing on whether the drugs worked — something already established — the researchers were charged with looking at something more subjective — how were the patients "feeling" and whether that feeling resulted in better compliance. It was an important distinction, businesswise as well, because doctors were more willing to write prescriptions for drugs that didn't generate patient complaints, as did traditional diuretics. The study employed prestigious researchers, from Harvard, Stanford, the London School of Hygiene, and Boston University, and its conclusions were striking. For the first time, statistical techniques were used to measure quality of life, and in three highly emotional areas of patient experience — work, exercise, and sexual performance — Capoten was superior. Consequently, patients taking it, in comparison to diuretics, were 40 to 60 percent less likely to stop taking the drug. In other words, they were not complaining to doctors. Capoten could be the physician's friend.

The study was published in the *New England Journal of Medi-*

cine, and almost immediately Squibb's stock price jumped 5 percent. Leschly brilliantly exploited the findings in medical journal advertising and promo pieces for the sales force. It was true that there were significant gaps in the study — Capoten should have been compared with all existing (and cheaper) antihypertensives, a charge that would come back to haunt the industry in later years, when cost became a factor. But the data were clear on the issue of "quality of life." The phrase itself was a perfect evocation of the 1980s ethos. As such it lent itself to the more creative forces in medical journal advertising: Capoten provided "expanded prescribing freedom." Doctors didn't have to monitor patients as closely for compliance. With Capoten, another journal ad said, "It appears that for the first time ever a patient can feel as well on treatment as he does off it." Quality of life is what mattered — it meant "a job well done," one ad proclaimed, invoking the notion of better performance at the office. "We spend so much of our lives at work," it went on, "performance is a key to our quality of life." In another ad depicting an attractive fiftyish couple at the beach, smiling as if ready to bonk at any moment, the copy proclaimed, "Quality of life means a feeling of well-being" (the drug had never been tested as a mood stabilizer or enhancer) and that quality of life "means sharing love."

Love! Business soared. By 1987, Capoten sales topped $700 million; that same year Squibb became the fastest-growing pharmaceuticals company in the world. In 1989, Capoten was a billion-dollar blockbuster.

For Leschly, the triumph was short-lived. All the aggressiveness, the exhortations to break the mold and keep score — such traits may have charmed the sales force but not fellow executives in Squibb's inner sanctum. Save for Furlaud, whom he often tutored in tennis, the top brass regarded Leschly as secretive, divisive, and even underhanded in his dealings with fellow management. That limited him as a possible successor to Furlaud, who, unknown to Leschly, had quietly begun considering a merger of Squibb with the much larger Bristol-Myers. In late 1989, Furlaud announced that he was indeed merging with Bristol, and that, in keeping with the fact of Squibb's relatively smaller size, he would be assuming the presidency of its pharmaceutical operations — essentially taking Leschly's job. Seeing no possibility of emerging on top — his dream — Leschly resigned.

For a year or so, he was rarely seen in the leafy New Jersey suburb where he lived. He enrolled in a graduate program in philosophy at Princeton University to take some time to think. There he came in contact with a number of American executives doing the same thing, rethinking what they were doing in life and in business — rethinking, in essence, what was important.

When Leschly left academia in 1990 and was hired to head the worldwide prescription-drug division of SmithKline Beecham, there were few outward signs that the Leschly style had changed. As his new right-hand man, Jean-Paul Garnier, told the *Wall Street Journal*, Leschly was making SmithKline into a company with "an extreme tolerance for mavericks. There is no clone, no mold, and though dealing with mavericks with very healthy egos doesn't make life any easier, they're encouraged here."

Yet the brief sojourn among his peers at Princeton had changed one thing about Leschly's priorities. No longer was he simply interested in marketing pills to physicians; he was interested in "the complete delivery of pharmaceutical care." By that he meant getting a piece of the managed care business. To do so he purchased a pharmaceuticals benefit manager (PBM), a firm that contracted with HMOs and managed care to get the best price for drugs and then to deliver them to the consumer via mail order and large institutional pharmacies. It was a decision fraught with antitrust perils, but Leschly believed he could hurdle such obstacles. He also invested $125 million in the emerging science of pharmacogenomics, the use of data from the Human Genome Project to target genes that caused illness.

The two undertakings became near obsessions. Increasingly Leschly saw pills not as chemicals but as software — and he saw that analogy as a way to justify the prices he had to charge. He often explained it to visiting analysts and journalists by rendering a version of a conversation he had with his mother: "Suddenly information technology was so essential that we realized we are an information company more than we are a pill company. Be-

cause it's the software — all the research, networking, marketing — that's important in that pill. The pill is a piece of software!
I mean, when my mother would ask, 'Why is that pill so expensive?' I would say, 'But, Ma, it's not the pill that costs so much,
it's the software!'" And if it was information — not pills — that
lay at the core of SmithKline, why, he would also have to recast
his own role. As he told a group of fellow CEOs at a Harvard
roundtable, "I'm restructuring my work habits. I now spend
about ninety percent of my time on strategic issues and ten percent on operational issues. I am almost totally disengaged from
day-to-day, tactical implementation."

And yet, for all the noise, by 1996 there was little in the way of
music from Leschly's two grand obsessions. The PBM business
was proving to be more complicated than it first looked, as well
as costlier to run. The genomic initiative held promise — and
held and held and held, perhaps until the next millennium, not
something about which the board of directors, itself constantly
fending off takeover battles, was particularly happy.

There was one saving grace — one old-style pill that might rescue the Leschly legacy. It was an antidepressant called paroxetine, brand name Paxil. SmithKline had acquired it in its merger
with the British pharmaceuticals firm Beecham in 1990. Like
many of the new-era drugs for treating mood disorders — Lilly's
Prozac was the model — Paxil was a chemical that did two
things, in varying degrees, in different individuals. It stimulated
some neurotransmitters, or brain chemicals, and that resulted in
some relief from depression. It also tranquilized other neuro-
chemical processes, leading to relief from anxiety for others.
Like Prozac and other similar chemicals, it was not much better
than the previous generation of antidepressants, or mood stabi-
lizers, but it did have one big thing, marketing-wise, in its favor:
it was almost impossible to overdose from it, and that made selling it to general practitioners, until then uneasy about prescribing psychiatric drugs for fear of such complications, a snap. This
feature created a huge new prescribing base.

Paxil was also, like Prozac, a powerful cultural product perfectly tailored to a generation of young men and women who

were not so keen on taking a pill simply to alter their mood; in the back of everyone's mind was the bad experience with Valium in the late 1970s, when thousands discovered they were hooked on something that was not supposed to be addictive. SmithKline got around that opprobrium the same way Prozac had — by focusing its marketing department on the telling of a "story." The story, often illustrated with brightly colored diagrams and cartoon characters, unfolded thus: Paxil worked on a different brain chemical system than did older drugs. The name of this "natural" brain chemical was serotonin. In some depressed patients, this chemical was lowered in volume because a certain brain synapse was "overactive," hoovering up too much of it. Paxil, by "naturally" blocking this too fervent neuro–vacuum cleaner, led to increased serotonin in the depressed and led — *voilà* — to relief from the depression. It was all a matter of restoring a natural balance.

It was true that every discrete action described in the reuptake–chemical balance story had some element of truth, some more so than others. But in the end, they were only theories. No one knew what serotonin balance was. It had rarely been measured (and when it had been measured it had been measured in dead people), and it would certainly never be measured in any patient coming to a general practitioner for a pill (the procedure involved a spinal tap). What *was* known was that both low *and* high levels of serotonin were associated with depression in different populations. Yet none of this really mattered. Paxil seemed to relieve depression in many people; the story simply helped resistant physicians explain the drug to reluctant patients. Some might view this subterfuge as fraud, but such was not a view heard very loudly in pharmaceutical or regulatory circles.

From the beginning, Paxil seemed to catch a disproportionate number of regulatory breaks. At the FDA, under new pressure to review drugs faster, Paxil sailed through. True, there were early concerns that the drug had its own unique addictive qualities, perhaps not as bad as Valium but certainly troublesome. Yet there was no FDA interest in the subject. Perhaps even more disturbing — albeit not to SmithKline — was the FDA's lack of interest in a small but very serious charge: that Paxil might be implicated, like Prozac, in increased suicides and suicide attempts. The agency attitude was documented in an internal SmithKline "FDA Conversation Record," in which the company's regulatory affairs chief, Thomas E. Donnelly, reported a discussion he had with Dr. Martin Brecher, then in the FDA's division of neuropharmacological drug products. "[Brecher] said that the public press has been widely discussing the relationship between fluoxetine (Prozac) and violence-ideation and suicide-ideation. Although the [FDA] division does not see it as a real issue, but as a public relations problem, Lilly has been asked to submit a detailed response to the public's concern. He is therefore asking that we do the same since we have a drug with a similar mechanism of action. He said his request is not based on any concern he has developed from his review of paroxetine." Of course, that lack of concern might have come about because SmithKline, like Lilly, had tweaked the data to make the drug look more benign than it was — or so some critics said. But such warnings simply did not resonate at the new "clientized" FDA. Paxil was approved for sale in the United States in early 1993.

Leschly was almost giddy with excitement. He called a meeting of his senior marketing people and laid out the sales strategy. The drug had great potential, he said, but the company was being too shy about promoting it. "We need to set some stretch goals," he said. The attitude had to be "We'll beat Pfizer — we'll beat Prozac!" He went on: "Look, if you ask for $3 billion in sales, you have a chance for $1.5 billion. But if you just ask for $1 billion, you will never get more than half a billion — so that's what I want the attitude for Paxil to be." The whole idea was to have "strategic intent," he said, harkening back to his young days in tennis. "I mean, look, when I was a kid my personal goal was always to be at Wimbledon. I didn't know how I was going to get there, but I always envisioned it — I would always smell the grass and hear the crowd — and that drove me. Same with this company!"

People who are not in sales love to make fun of such talk; it all sounds so jockish, so boys-clubbish, and, frankly, so mendacious. But in the corporate context, even in the most open big-business culture, candid expressions of big goals by the head guy are rare. They are, in fact, craved, particularly by the sales department, the frontline warriors, who feed on the stimulation and attention. At SmithKline the exhortations produced the desired effect. Paxil sales soared.

The Leschly effect proved especially popular in the marketing department. That division had gotten word from the company's pharmacologists that Paxil was "selective." To pharmacologists, this meant that the drug did not act on *all* neurotransmitter systems. What the marketing department heard was simply that it was "selective," connoting some kind of "cleanness" in the way it acted on the body, again a valuable way to distinguish it from a previous generation of "dirty" drugs. Thus was born the notion of a selective serotonin reuptake inhibitor, or SSRI. It really meant nothing in practice, particularly to the general practitioner, who rarely (if ever) read journals on psychopharmacology. But it did make Paxil seem, somehow, better. The department promptly commissioned a series of now famous ads, using a pool table, to demonstrate how other antidepressants were "scattershot" and how Paxil was a clean, clear eight ball in the side pocket.

But by 1995, Paxil was still not reaching Leschly's stretch goals. There were persistent reports that it caused a withdrawal reaction; in fact, withdrawal syndrome was the number one reported adverse effect, something noted by both SmithKline and the FDA. The company attempted to deal with the issue by ignoring it, relabeling Paxil eleven times and relegating the withdrawal reaction to a less prominent part of the label. It didn't work. Media reports persisted.

But Leschly's product development group had a new stretch plan. Instead of trying to hit its goal by selling Paxil as an antidepressant, why not enlarge the base by selling it as a cure for a number of related psychiatric disorders? In other words, why not view it as a drug that did many things, rather than narrowly as a cure for one disease? There was, for example, the notion of a "panic" disorder, a highly agitated state set off by both specific and nonspecific circumstances; among psychiatrists there was little agreement about what panic disorder really was, except that, at one time, they used to prescribe Valium for it. There was also a better-studied phenomenon, obsessive-compulsive disorder, or OCD; like "panic" there had been no new treatments for it for decades. It was true that real OCD was very rare; most psychiatrists' training told them that they would be lucky if they saw a single true case of OCD once in their entire careers. But this did not inhibit Leschly's marketing department either. Why not exploit Paxil's similarities to the old drugs — only the good ones, that is — and apply to the FDA for a new indication for panic and OCD? That would create whole new markets. After all, people who used to take Valium but didn't like using a drug that was called a tranquilizer still needed to be medicated, didn't they?

And there was one other opportunity, a phenomenon known as social phobia disorder. Like OCD it was a bona fide psychiatric disease, a debilitating lack of social confidence that led its sufferers to lives of isolation, loneliness, and inability to perform many of the simplest tasks of everyday life. In small studies, people diagnosed with the disorder responded to Paxil favorably; it calmed them down. The trouble was that true social phobia disorder was rare. Very rare. It affected, at least as traditionally measured, very few people in the United States or Europe. It was mainly known as "an Asian disorder." But SmithKline's marketing department determined that that might have been because people who were so shy did not come forward for diagnosis.

To set the stage for Paxil's social phobia launch, Leschly's marketing department went to work, commissioning a huge publicity campaign to raise awareness of the disease. In many ways, the effort cut the pattern for many to follow, both by SmithKline and its competitors: Hire a public relations agency to produce a free video on the disease and distribute it widely for use by network affiliates and independent TV stations, who were always starved for health stories (especially free health stories). Underwrite studies by experts in the field, who conclude that the disorder is debilitating and probably afflicts many more people than previously supposed. Detail with graphics and personal stories about how social phobia, or, as SmithKline recast the name, social anxiety disorder (SAD), wreaked havoc on workplace productivity and sexual satisfaction.

As the SAD campaign got under way, a new opportunity arose — the growing awareness, partly driven by the industry itself, of child and adolescent depression, again a real disease but one that few general practitioners felt comfortable treating with drugs. And again, in some very preliminary studies, youngsters seemed to respond to Paxil. To pave the way for a hoped-for FDA approval, SmithKline began underwriting clinical trials and then distributing the data at various pediatric forums. There were small voices that cried alarm, citing the thinness of the data and the fear that such de facto off-label promotion might lead to overprescribing by general practitioners who had no clue how to treat the disease. But by now the climate had changed; the Supreme Court had said that drug companies had the right to distribute such data. To complain that they shouldn't was simply patronizing, and we couldn't have any of that.

By 2000, the divide-and-stretch strategy had worked brilliantly; Paxil was now approved for depression, panic disorder, obsessive-compulsive disorder, and social anxiety disorder, which commentators routinely described on nightly TV as affecting "ten million in the United States alone." Many in the company believed an indication for childhood depression was right around the corner; general practitioners, after all, were already prescribing the drug to children. By the end of 2000, Paxil had sales exceeding $2.1 billion, and there was no end in sight for new indications.

Despite that success, analysts were not strong on SmithKline Beecham stock. Leschly may have done a good job by mining one or two drugs for their enormous potential, but he had been a failure at developing a pipeline of promising new drugs that would take Paxil's place when it came off patent. Instead he had gone on tangents — the Human Genome Project was one example, the failed PBM venture another. Now whenever people heard him talk, it wasn't about new drugs but about the Internet, about how the Web was going to change everything and how big pharma had to be a part of that. On the Web, he said, people would have instant access to all of their health information, and SmithKline could play the role of a "health partner." He could see it now, he would tell anyone who would listen: "The whole world is changing! Now the patient has the information. He will be a partner with SmithKline and his doctor. If you are a diabetic, and that really bugs you, *really gets under your skin*, well, you will spend hours a month studying up on it. Forty percent of the Net is people seeking health information, and we are going to be there. Now the patient has the information, and they will demand transparency. They will demand control. They can go to any site and dig in and get very quality information, get the answer, print it out, go to your physician, and the physician says, 'Wow, yeah, I just heard about this from SmithKline!'"

While Leschly certainly would have warmed the hearts of the folks at the Washington Legal Foundation, he was not exactly getting a wow at SmithKline, which in late 2001 was taken over by the British firm Glaxo. Sir Richard Sykes, Glaxo's chairman, did not get along with Leschly, and, like Furlaud a decade before at Squibb, he had no problem with edging him out. At the new company, GlaxoSmithKline, they had other priorities, and Jan Leschly's brand of blue-skying was not one of them. In the new world of pharmaceutical leadership, if you spouted big paradigm-busting ideas, they'd better pay off — fast.

THE CREATION OF CHRONIC DISEASE

Glaxo, the pharmaceuticals giant that ate Jan Leschly, had been small game only two decades earlier. In the boggy pharma jungle, it swung on the vine of prior greatness while withering on stultifying British business practices. It was not always thus: Glaxo began life as a vibrant trading company in mid-nineteenth-century London. In the early 1900s, it began manufacturing dried milk, eventually emerging as the United Kingdom's principal purveyor of baby formula, food, and vitamins. After WWII, the firm got into pharmaceuticals. Some of its hits were B_{12} for pernicious anemia, streptomycin for TB treatment, and albuterol for asthma. It was, by the late 1970s, a middling, predictable player — one that its president, an intense, enterprising man named Paul Girolamo, believed was ready to jump to the next rung of competition.

The reason for Girolamo's optimism was a new Glaxo drug called ranitidine, or Zantac. Zantac was one of only two new drugs (the other was SmithKline's Tagamet, or cimetidine) approved to treat ulcers. The drugs, called H2 blockers, worked by inhibiting the expression of histamines, body chemicals that drive up stomach acid, then believed to be the cause of ulcer sores. The market was huge, and the company had spent an enormous amount of money on the drug. But two things were deeply wrong. One, there was no way that the British and continental markets would give Glaxo the payoff it needed in terms of Zantac sales; the regulatory processes and the health care systems in those countries were slow, slow, slow. And so were European consumers, at least when it came to demanding drugs for gastrointestinal ailments.

The other problem was the competition. SmithKline had managed to drive Tagamet onto the market first, in 1976, and it was establishing hegemony in many countries. After a long wrangle with his fussy U.K. board, Girolamo decided that there was only one way to deal with Tagamet — get into the fray in the United States, the rival drug's home turf, where there were some 10 million ulcer sufferers. It was not a hard case to marshal; after all, at the time Glaxo had more sales in Nigeria than in the United States, then as now the world's richest market for pills. The board concurred. Girolamo purchased a Florida vitamin company as a corporate shell for Glaxo's American headquarters, and, in 1981, launched Zantac in the United States. By 1985, he had managed to capture a significant portion of new anti-ulcer prescriptions, but he still lagged far behind his ambition, which he liked to state in the negative: "If there is one failure it is that Tagamet exists at all." And to take care of that, he needed an American, not another Brit.

Fortunately, one was available. His name was Ernest Mario. The son of a New Jersey janitor, Mario was a classic by-his-own-bootstraps success story, muscling himself through the pharma ranks until landing at Squibb, where he flourished as an executive. In 1985, Girolamo, acting on a tip from a former Squibb executive, went poaching. He promptly hired Mario as the one to go out and shoot down Tagamet for Glaxo.

This Mario did with efficiency and relish. He tripled the sales force and pushed it to detail hospitals and physicians about the superiority of Zantac over Tagamet. This endeavor was tricky; if the FDA is clear about one thing when it comes to promotion, it is any claim of therapeutic or safety superiority. Such claims are costly and difficult, if not impossible, to prove, and Zantac had few studies to buttress its case. But by the late 1980s, even before the Court's sanction of off-label, a good detail person was adept at toeing that line, and Mario invested heavily in recruiting and training exactly that kind of salesperson. He spun out new off-label promotions, a low-dose formulation for use by children and another to "prevent" ulcers from recurring. The strategy worked; in 1989, Zantac toppled Tagamet.

Mario then pushed Glaxo's research and development department to come up with a new raft of drugs, for when Zantac came off patent. Many of them were compounds that acted on the neurotransmitter serotonin. One, known as GR 38032, blocked vomiting "messages" sent to the gut by serotonin and could be valuable in cancer therapy. Another compound that mimicked serotonin, GR 43175, might be good for treating migraines. There were also new candidates for asthma and depression. The guiding light, regardless of therapeutic potential, however, was clear and simple: All of the new drugs had to have potential sales of $180 million or more. Drugs that would bring in revenues of $50 million a year or less "would be crazy. It would cost us more than that to develop them."

Yet all of these plans rested on the continued success of Zantac, then making up about a third of all Glaxo revenue. This hope was far from assured. Not only was Merck, the King Kong of the U.S. pharmaceuticals world, readying its own new anti-ulcer medication, but there was also, for Mario, disturbing news coming from the world of medical science. Ever since 1984, researchers studying the causes of ulcers had focused not on stomach acid, upon which Zantac acted, but on bacteria. Australian researchers were showing how one such bug, *Heliobacter pylori*, was present in as many as 90 percent of patients with duodenal ulcers and in 70 percent of those with gastric ulcers. The implication, hopeful for ulcer patients, was also dismal for Glaxo. It wasn't an increase in stomach acid that was the problem, the problem Zantac treated so well. It was bacteria, which could be treated instead with an antibiotic. The negative sales implications were huge, and for years Glaxo (and mainstream U.S. pharma scientists) both privately and publicly pooh-poohed the *Heliobacter* theory, stressing the idiosyncratic nature of ulcers. But by the early 1990s, with some of the first studies of antibiotic treatment of ulcers appearing, the Grim Reaper had come for Zantac. If it were to remain a big cash cow — as the company required it to be — it would have to be repositioned for a bigger market.

Again, Mario and his retooled American staff went back to basics: What did Zantac do, and whom would it benefit? The answer came in the form of a disease that almost no one ever got: GERD, short for gastroesophageal reflux disease. GERD is, in essence, heartburn that gets so bad and so chronic that it causes damage to the esophagus. True GERD is rare, but the precondition for it, a weak esophageal sphincter (the muscle that shuts off the esophagus from lower gut acids) is part of the natural aging process. That is why almost everyone gets heartburn, and why almost everyone's heartburn gets worse with age. The business question was: How could you convince a lot of people — and a lot of physicians and insurers — to pay for an expensive prescription drug when most people saw heartburn in a benign way and treated it with a 49-cent roll of Tums? Worse, from the perspective of the CEO, much of the resistance to any anti-GERD medication was populist, the outgrowth of long-held folk wisdom: people felt that heartburn was, at least in part, their own fault, either from eating too much or from eating the wrong foods at the wrong time. How could you sell around that?

The answer was to medicalize — and by extension popularize

— GERD. Although, to its credit, Glaxo funded a broad spectrum of therapeutic information initiatives, the new mission was as clear as a bell: create public awareness of GERD and brand Zantac as its cure. As Irwin C. Gerson, the lead advertising account executive who brainstormed the graphic of an erupting volcano to drive home the graveness of the "disease," later admitted, "GERD is heartburn."

The tactic worked so well — sending Zantac sales into the heavens — that it has since become a textbook example of what the industry now routinely called "branding a condition." As *Medical Marketing and Media* described it in a hortatory March 2003 review,

> GERD elevated the medical importance of this condition by presenting it as an acutely chronic "disorder" with the underlying physiological etiology and the potential for serious long-term consequences if left untreated — a far cry from the "plop plop fizz fizz" perception of heartburn. The company launched a well-coordinated initiative by creating the Glaxo Institute for Digestive Health (GIDH), which served as a platform for education and awareness. The GIDH sponsored research awards in the area of GI health, discussed GERD in the context of other serious gastrointestinal diseases, involved powerful third-party advocates such as the American College of Gastroenterology and fielded a public relations effort called Heartburn Across America.

The results: "Not only did GSK double the percentage of physicians who perceived them as leaders in GI health, but helped to drive annual sales of Zantac to over $2 billion at peak, 65 percent of which was accounted for by GERD." By 1992, when Mario was named CEO of Glaxo's worldwide holdings company, Zantac made up 44 percent of the company's bottom line.

There were, of course, the typical party poopers, inevitable at any pharma victory celebration. As GERD prescriptions soared, a number of gastroenterologists wondered, albeit briefly, what it would mean for an entire population routinely to suppress its natural stomach acid production for long periods of time, merely to treat their imprudent lifestyle choices. Such voices fell mute when met with the counterclaim, underwritten by Glaxo, that they were blaming the victim. Others worried about the medical consequences of long-term *low* stomach acid, particularly since low stomach acid was a problem in old age, when more acid is needed to aid in the breakdown of vital nutrients. Again, there was no market for such a voice, and so that voice quickly disappeared into the GERD chorus.

THE CREATION OF HEALTH

It says something about the transitive, fugitive nature of success in the modern pharma CEO suite that, not long after the triumph of GERD, came the fall of Ernest Mario. For reasons never officially proffered, Mario left Glaxo in 1993, just as his U.S. operation became the driving force for the whole company. His ouster was likely political; his aggressive manner of pushing Zantac for unapproved uses had earned Glaxo a number of warning letters from the FDA, and with the Clinton administration talking up the idea (quickly batted down by allegedly more sober minds) of price controls on prescription drugs, that was something that London could certainly do without. From a realpolitik view, Glaxo's board may have decided that enough had been gained from having a gunslinger; Tagamet was not dead but it was badly wounded. And now, with Glaxo moving into the top ranks, it might be time for a less aggressive-*appearing* executive. And its board had just the fellow in mind. In late 1993, it named Robert Ingram as executive over Glaxo's American operations.

It was an inspired choice, because Ingram, an upbeat, congenial man with a fondness for NASCAR racing, was state-of-the-art when it came to pharma executives, a true hybrid of the political and marketing species. Ingram began his career in sales at Merrill-Dow, where he climbed the greasy pole to head public affairs and later governmental affairs. It was at Merrill that Ingram was exposed to the powerful potential of direct-to-consumer advertising and marketing. In 1983 he commissioned a study of five hundred viewers of Cable Health Network who saw a thirty-second commercial about the effects of cholesterol. The results:

two weeks after seeing the ad, 22 percent had visited their doctors, and 46 percent of those asked to have their cholesterol checked. As the study authors told Ingram in an internal memo, "These results are nothing less than staggering." Ingram took the advice to heart. He was one of the few respondents to John Dingell's 1984 inquisition who did not favor an outright ban on DTC. There was another formative experience as well. Later, at Glaxo, where prior to being named chief he had been laboring in the trenches of administrative and regulatory affairs since 1990, Ingram had witnessed Mario's rise and fall. The lesson was that successful pharma executives had to invest in regulatory savvy — smart, specialized ways to communicate with government regulators — as well as marketing and science.

Ingram was, to be sure, a charismatic man as well, easily fitting into Glaxo's U.S. culture, in Yoo-hoo-drinking Raleigh-Durham, where the company built its slick new U.S. headquarters. He was brainy and given to synthesis. As Glaxo's new drugs began to come onto the market, first the antivomiting medications, then new compounds for asthma, AIDS, depression, irritable bowel syndrome, genital herpes, back pain and chronic pain and hypertension — the whole raft of aging boomer concerns — Ingram began to see what he liked to call a "new pharmaceutical paradigm." This he loved to talk about, first in small company staff meetings, later at big pharma conferences. Selling pills was no longer just about curing a disease, he said. It was about "creating a state of health." It was important to frame it this way, Ingram said, because, more and more, big pharma was being asked to justify its choices: Why should there be another antidepressant? Why should it cost so much? You could not cure depression, after all, just as you could not cure allergies or asthma or cancer or AIDS. "But already today, and I believe even more so in the future, we are delivering both a cure and products and services that add to the quality of life," he proclaimed in one speech. "In some cases, we are replacing a disease state with a healthy state." He liked to cite the example of AIDS, where "combination therapies are knocking back the viral load in many patients to limits undetectable by our most sophisticated tests."

Perhaps the best example of the new paradigm was a drug called bupropion, branded as Wellbutrin. Glaxo had acquired the compound from another firm, intending to market it as an antidepressant. But early test marketing indicated that Wellbutrin produced unanticipated seizures in a small population of patients; even when the company fixed the problem by changing the dosage, doctors were reluctant to prescribe it. The first impression, however unfair, had stuck. So Ingram commissioned a series of studies to show that Wellbutrin was not only safe, but had fewer side effects than the SSRIs being hawked by Lilly, Pfizer, and SmithKline, with far less sexual dysfunction. He then discharged a corps of medical advisers — essentially salesmen with medical training or even M.D. degrees — to chat up leading mental health specialists, whose prescribing patterns are closely tracked by fellow experts. The tactic worked, and Wellbutrin soon took its place in the apothecary of modern psychopharmacology. Ingram also caught a break when physicians at a local veterans hospital found that depressed vets put on Wellbutrin were more likely to stop smoking. For them it created a whole new state of health! That allowed Glaxo to win another indication for the drug, beefing up Ingram's arsenal of health creation.

In all of this activity, Ingram was learning one thing: it didn't matter how good your drug was if doctors didn't know about it, or if they had gotten a bad first impression. Somehow you had to find a way to control that first impression — and then reinforce it. After all, he could not afford to respin every drug, as he had done with Wellbutrin; that was simply not cost-effective. Nor was the traditional method of going on a hiring binge and carpet-bombing doctors' offices with sales reps. By the mid-nineties, every single major pharmaceutical company had done that. There were now 80,000 pharma reps nationwide. Tales abounded at sales conferences about how there were so many sales reps waiting in hospital parking lots that it was not uncommon for a Lilly rep on his way out to, literally, rear-end a Pfizer rep who was on her way in. And, almost as bad, the FDA was cracking down again on just what reps could and could not say, something that irked the former regulatory affairs man in Ingram. He decided there had to be a better way.

The better way came via Ingram's marketing department. Instead of spending the entire promotions budget on sales calls, they would spend some of it on "closed circuit computer detailing." That would allow the company to deliver, from headquarters, very targeted information to leading "high writers" — physicians who controlled lots of patients for specific diseases at high-profile institutions. For physicians, there was a tangible incentive. Every physician who signed up would get a free audio-video-equipped computer in return for entering a three-year contract agreeing to accept, during business hours, one video-conference sales session with a Glaxo rep every month. It was, in essence, a way to buy face time.

But just what went on during such a session? Typically, as I observed in a morning spent at Glaxo's customer response center, it worked like this: John Dalpe, a thirteen-year sales veteran, would dial up a physician who was "on the program," as he put it. On this morning he was on the program with a Dr. Milgram, a specialist in asthma and allergies at a huge San Diego hospital. After querying her about whether she had been prescribing one of Glaxo's respiratory products, he pulled up on his screen, unbeknownst to her, data that characterized her prescriptions for the past six months. Flonase, the company's newest allergy spray, seemed to lag. He asked Milgram about it, and the pair had a leisurely conversation; there was no hard sell. No patient names were used, of course, but as Dalpe explained to me later, "This is a powerful sales tool." To demonstrate, he pulled up a promotional sheet on Flonase. "See? I can talk to her about this and then draw circles around the areas I really want her to read. That's a great thing," he went on, "because you can't do that in [hard] type without running afoul of FDA regs. But because she can't print this out, I can — and she can get the benefits of the latest research."

There was, of course, another way to read this win-win scenario. Glaxo was getting *too* good at beating the regulatory process. One example was Ingram's response to an FDA advisory panel's assessment of a new Glaxo drug to treat influenza, Relenza, which the company billed as a way to cut the length of flu symptoms to seventy-two hours. Glaxo had submitted three studies showing the drug's efficacy. The results were, at best, mixed. Then a young FDA reviewer, Michael Elashoff, dug more deeply into the data. What he found was remarkable. Only one study had been conducted in the United States, and that data was the weakest. When you corrected for all of the study's epidemiological lapses and inconsistencies, he said, Relenza was a wash; it did almost nothing for sick Americans, who tended to take more OTC medications for the flu and so, unlike the patients in the foreign studies, did not respond as robustly to the drug. Elashoff made a pointed, compelling presentation to the Anti-Viral Drugs Advisory Committee, detailing the flaws and showing how the drug caused dangerous bronchospasm in the elderly, the very population Ingram had positioned Relenza to serve. He then drove the stake in by concluding that "more Relenza patients compared to placebo patients had a recurrence of the symptoms." The committee voted against approval of Relenza. Although advisory committee recommendations are just that, the FDA often follows the advice.

Ingram was outraged. Quickly he had his regulatory lawyers draw up a lengthy response and sent it to the FDA chief. What was remarkable was the personal nature of the thirty-three-page letter. It named Elashoff thirty times as someone who had misinterpreted its data. "The fact is," Ingram explained in an interview, "this was an advisory committee meeting where one statistician took the balance of the discussion *in the wrong direction!* I mean, we looked at the rules and they were clear: We had two double-blind studies that showed efficacy and safety, so we should have an approvable drug! We actually had three, eh, but the third just showed a lesser benefit."

The letter worked. For reasons never stated, and with no response to Elashoff's damning analysis, the FDA approved Relenza in time for flu season in 1999. Almost immediately Elashoff's FDA career plunged. "I was told I wouldn't be doing any more advisory committee meetings, I wouldn't be working on any drugs that were quote unquote controversial. And there was the suggestion, it's probably better if you leave the division." A few months later he left the FDA for a position in a genetic research company.

But Glaxo and Ingram had learned a valuable lesson: the new FDA, she read the mail, and she listened to agile regulatory wonks.

Nothing drove this home to the company as did the experience with another new drug, Lotronex, for irritable bowel syndrome. IBS, as it is known, is a chronic disease that, because it causes unremitting diarrhea, mainly in women, can be truly disabling. Lotronex, via its ability to inhibit the processes that cause diarrhea, was a promising compound, with one clinical trial showing its benefits. It was approved in June 1999. Almost immediately concerns surfaced about Lotronex's safety; once released into a large and eager population, most of whom, unlike the test population, were largely unmonitored by their physicians, the drug started doing unanticipated things. Reports from patients, hospitals, and physicians indicated that Lotronex caused ischemic colitis — constipation that was so profound as to become life-threatening — and led several FDA scientists to recommend that the drug be recalled. But Glaxo believed that the side effects could be ameliorated with a recommendation for increased physician monitoring. In the midsummer of 2000, the company sent a team of "reg affairs" people to the FDA to make their case. They prevailed. Instead of recalling the drug, the FDA simply issued a medication management guideline. Despite the guideline's failure to address the FDA scientists' concerns — that "pain" as a symptom that something was going wrong was a symptom that came too late in the potentially fatal ischemic colitis process to do anyone any good — Lotronex would stay on the market.

Three months later, after five patients died and dozens more were admitted to emergency rooms for ruptured bowels, Glaxo withdrew the drug from the market.

Yet right away its reg affairs people began working on a way to get it back on the market, which they succeeded in doing by mid-2002. It was, for everyone in the company's executive suite, another regulatory victory. The company's stock continued to soar. By 2003, Glaxo, now merged with SmithKline (a process begun in 2000), was the second largest pharmaceuticals company in the world.

CIRCUS OF SYNERGY

In 1994, Merck, the grand old daddy of American pharma, committed what it once might have considered pure heresy: it hired someone from outside its ranks to head the company. It was a move almost entirely designed to meet a new pharma dilemma: managed care.

Managed care companies, with their lock on the health care spending of most big firms, were proving fierce negotiators over the price of pills — something the industry had never had to confront. Slowly but surely — and it didn't take an advanced degree in accounting or forecasting to fathom — such negotiating was coming right out of the hide of big pharma. The managed care phenomenon cut hard another way: now consumers, once known as patients, were restive over the issue of price. They too were getting hit with cuts — cuts in the amount most health insurance plans would pay for care, including pills. In his first term, Bill Clinton picked up on the mood and began hinting at price controls on drugs and, perhaps, a Medicare drug benefit — something big pharma hated because it brought with it the specter of even more hardball price negotiators. At Merck, the new pressure on price had arrived as a storm. Only a few years before, Merck, which had been touted as "the miracle company," was now, as *Business Week* pronounced, "showing its age."

Raymond Gilmartin, the man the board eventually hired to slow the aging process, was in almost every way his predecessor's alter ego. Roy Vagelos, the outgoing CEO, had been a scholar, a brilliant NIH scientist, and a veteran drug developer in his own right, responsible for shepherding through the world's first statin. He was a science-first kind of guy, constantly invoking the company's high-minded commitment to original research. Gilmartin was an engineer by education, a salesman by inclination. He had been CEO of a successful, if unsexy, company that made medical devices. At Merck it was clear he had no problem cutting costs and focusing on the pragmatic issues at hand. If a line of research was going nowhere, it was time to shut off its lights. If layoffs were in order, so be it. To the Merck board, Gilmartin was the perfect antidote to Vagelos, in substance and even in style. Where Vagelos had grown aloof, and, in his later years, highhanded, Gilmartin was congenial, down-to-earth; he was your laconic but kindly Irish uncle who always brought you the best present at holiday time. In Merck, Gilmartin himself found a midcareer apotheosis. He was, he said, "exhilarated."

His predecessor had left him one untapped legacy: a company called Medco, one of the hottest health care companies going. Medco did not make drugs, and it did not deliver any form of medical care. In the new health care economy, Medco was a go-between. For a fee, it negotiated with pharma companies on behalf of huge managed care plans controlled by corporations and unions. Leveraging such huge purchasing power allowed Medco to get discounts not afforded to other pharma customers. Medco then passed on the discount, usually via bulk and individual mail order sales, to its clients' employees. It was a profitable company. The firm had grown from $20 million in annual sales in 1983 to $2.2 billion in 1993. And it had done so by taking giant bites out of big pharma, Merck included. It was true that there was a "slight" antitrust issue in Merck owning the company: Medco's first allegiance, at least in negotiations over drug prices, was not, in theory and in law, to Merck. It was to the customer. Just prior to Merck's acquisition, for example, Medco was urging doctors to shift from Merck's Mevacor to Squibb's Pravachol, for price reasons.

But Gilmartin did not see complexities and problems as much as he saw synergies and opportunities. In fact, as Gilmartin thumbed through the reports from various Merck divisions, what he found was not an empty drug pipeline, which many had imagined, but, rather, one that had not been adequately tended and plumbed. He quickly cut out unnecessary projects and focused the researchers almost entirely on drugs that treated chronic diseases. What he found was a rich vein. There were

Cozaar and Hyzaar, new antihypertensives that were better tolerated than the old generation. There was Fosamax, the first in a
new class of compounds that treated osteoporosis. There was
Singulair, a once-a-day asthma drug. He also leaned on the Merck
researchers to start thinking about clinical trials in a broader
way, to brainstorm ways to show tangible health outcomes from
the drugs; it wasn't enough to show that, for example, Zocor, the
new Merck statin, reduced cholesterol; they had to show that
it directly led to reduced heart attacks. Ditto a new drug like
Fosamax. "I pushed them to do extra research to show that not
only does it build bone density, but that it prevents breakages."
The force behind such moves was, again, the rising power of insurance companies and managed care, which insisted on seeing
evidence of the economic impact of new drugs. Did they save the
payer money in the form of reduced surgeries and hospitalizations or not?

Gilmartin imposed tightly circumscribed criteria for deciding
which drugs got the go-ahead for development: Was there a large
patient population? Was there a new pathway of disease that the
company understood and a novel mechanism of action that the
drug exploited in treating that pathway? Would patients tolerate
the drug well and be relatively free of side effects? And, equally
important, could it be delivered in a form that could be taken just
once a day? To the board he explained the new mantra: "What
matters here is how fast are you growing and how profitable are
you." Not how full is the pipeline, but how big and how fast will
your pipeline pay off?

If there was ever a drug that fit Ray Gilmartin's dream, it was
one known as L-748, 731, for treatment of arthritis pain. The
patient population was huge, by Merck's estimates as many as
40 million in the United States alone. Traditional drugs for
chronic pain, known as nonsteroidal anti-inflammatory drugs, or
NSAIDs, could be problematic; if you used them too often, they
could cause all kinds of gastrointestinal problems, including perforated ulcers and kidney failure. The reason was their design.
Pain is caused by the release of arachidonic acids after a cell is
damaged. Arachidonic acid is converted to another body chemi-

cal called prostaglandins, which have many effects: some cause inflammation and some maintain cellular structure in the gut. They are converted to those two functions by an enzyme system known as cyclooxygenase, COX. There are two COX systems, COX-1 and COX-2. In Merck's scenario, COX-1 is "good." It maintains protections against insults to the stomach lining by making the good prostaglandins; you do not want to inhibit COX-1. COX-2 is not so good. It stimulates the pain prostaglandin and the cascade of enzymes that cause the pain response. Traditional NSAIDs inhibit both COX systems, alleviating pain but also reducing the gut's ability to protect itself and thus causing many daily NSAID users to end up in the hospital with severe, sometimes life-threatening gastrointestinal injury.

The compound in Merck's Canadian labs, however, was selective. It did not inhibit COX-1, and as Gilmartin and his development executives saw it, such a COX-2 inhibitor would not only be profitable, but also conform to the new realities of pharmacoeconomics: you could prove that its health benefits also saved health care plans money because they would not be paying for stomach and kidney problems, which were expensive to treat. Gilmartin turned up the heat on the team responsible for L-748, 731, named rofecoxib, or Vioxx. Clinical trials of the drug in some five thousand patients were favorable, showing that Vioxx relieved pain not only in arthritics, but also after dental surgery and in women with severe menstrual pain. In that way it was just as good as a traditional NSAID. Then the team went further. Using an endoscope to examine the gastrointestinal tract of those patients, it was found that Vioxx was comparable to a placebo in terms of disturbance to the gut — on that count it was much better than traditional NSAIDs. There were, in the growing excitement about the drug, some concerns. There was a small increase in heart attacks among some who took it, and there were some who registered increased liver toxicity. But the coronaries were largely linked to the observation that the Vioxx patients were not taking aspirin anymore, which was linked with decreased heart attacks; it wasn't Vioxx that was the culprit, Merck insisted. And the liver toxicity was simply something that could be controlled by good physician monitoring.

This, of course, somewhat mitigated the drug's pharmaco-economic benefits, but that cavil fell on deaf ears. The FDA was convinced by Merck's trials, and in May 1999 the agency approved Vioxx. The company announced it as "one of the fastest drug development successes in the history of Merck & Co."

Speed, in fact, was quickly becoming the watchword at Merck. As the company itself explained to investors and the press, "The speed and skill with which Merck developed Vioxx was matched only by those of their American colleagues at the Merck Manufacturing Division. In the United States, just four days after FDA approval, the new medication was already being shipped to customers. Eleven days after approval, more than 30,000 pharmacies had shelves stocked with Vioxx." The media response was enormous; news shows proclaimed the drugs as "superaspirins" that would bring about the "end of pain." The networks followed, featuring lead stories in prime time (and DTC ads later in the evening). Sales boomed.

The Gilmartin way was working. Not only did it seem to work in the run-up and launch of Vioxx, a sexy drug by any measure, but also in the less glamorous compounds. Between 1995 and 2001, Merck launched seventeen new drugs, treating hypertension, elevated cholesterol, osteoporosis, male-pattern hair loss, GERD, acute pain, bacterial infection, and asthma. The company won approval for vaccines and medications for hepatitis, HIV infections, Parkinson's, and measles, but they remained relatively minor items in the portfolio. It was drugs for chronic conditions that received the overwhelming majority of Merck's research and marketing budgets. The temple of science, as the old-timers at Merck knew the company, was still a temple of science, but now the science was much more directed by the commercial imperative. To be fair, some of that was due to the rise of powerful institutional investors, who had come to rely on pharma's 20 percent annual earnings. Unlike Vagelos, Gilmartin instinctively understood this. He invested heavily in investor relations, using the Internet and regular investor advisories to keep the "community" informed of breakthroughs that would affect stock price.

There was also Medco, his predecessor Vagelos's gambit into

the arena of drug benefit management. Gilmartin saw the venture differently. Medco wasn't just going to be a separate cost and profit center, merely selling its pharmaceuticals benefit management service to big companies. "I saw it as a new mindset," Gilmartin explained. "It couldn't just be 'What would Medco do for Merck?' It had to be 'What could Merck do for Medco?'" Gilmartin saw that, just as the expectations for big pharma had changed, so too had expectations of a late-twentieth-century pharmaceuticals benefit manager. Clients like Ford and GM now expected companies like Medco to do more than merely negotiate good prices for pills and then mail them out to employees. They wanted PBMs to get into the new area of disease management — mainly by providing the consumer-patient with state-of-the-art information about medicine, how to "maintain medication compliance," and how to get the most out of the pills. They also wanted PBMs to engage patients on such subjects as personal health responsibilities — getting them to exercise more and eat better.

So Gilmartin invested heavily in upgrading Medco's technological database, allowing better communication with individual patients, helping them with disease management programs. He also transferred a large number of its traditional Merck medical personnel — M.D.s and Ph.D.s — to Medco, which allowed the subsidiary to help clients craft specialized health improvement plans for specific corporate populations. If General Motors saw that more and more of its health care money was being spent on treating heart disease, for example, Medco could craft special prevention and treatment plans, often mentioning Zocor and its rivals, as part of that plan, as well as sponsoring clinics for cholesterol screening and state-of-the-art information on healthful eating and exercise.

On the Internet, it was now easy for a patient who got her Vioxx from Medco to have her own personalized "health toolbox," where she might register all of her doctor appointments, medication times, and medication renewal dates. The Medco site would then prompt her to comply with her meds regimen, or to take her blood pressure, to go out and walk for thirty minutes, to weigh herself, and then enter the data so that she could "chart her improvements."

In this great circus of synergy, there remained, of course, the ongoing conflict of interest: Was Merck pushing Medco to favor its own products over lesser-priced rivals? There was preliminary evidence that the company was doing just that, but regulators at the time were not interested in the subject. The FTC, which governs such concerns, was largely quiescent, content to let the company regulate itself in exchange for written promises that it would not cross the line. To the few who pushed the issue, Gilmartin responded, "We will always have a policy of independence for Medco."

But Medco could do a lot more for Merck, particularly with its patient and physician data. Medco owned that data, and that information, collected directly from physicians and patients, could be used to paint demographic portraits of how certain populations prescribed and used prescription drugs. The patient information was anonymous; no names were attached to it, but it was highly specific about behavior and attributes. Through it a good marketing department could discern all kinds of things. One could perform sophisticated data mining to ferret out, say, all Medco physicians who were gynecologists who prescribed pain medications. Although Vioxx was not at the time approved for premenstrual pain, one of the primary complaints for which such a specialist might use such a drug, the data would show Merck marketers which ob-gyns were open to suggestion. How? By then doing a data-mining operation to sort out which ones were prescribing, say, Neurontin. That would tell the marketing people that these gynecologists were "innovators" (a less charitable term would be "experimenters") because Neurontin was approved only for epilepsy: Why else would the physician be prescribing it except for some off-label purpose, like pain? *Voilà:* the next time a Merck sales rep showed up to see that physician, he would bring along the latest study on Vioxx and premenstrual pain and mention that the physician might want to read it. Thus would the off-label "information" meet the off-label doctor meet the inevitable boxful of free samples.

Vioxx, Zocor, Singulair, Fosamax, Medco — by the year 2000, the mainstays of the Gilmartin way had transformed Merck. It was now as much an information company as it was a pill company. For stockholders, the upshot of that was best summarized in Merck's annual report: sales stood at $40.3 billion, up a stunning 23 percent from the previous year. Profits were even more impressive: the company cleared more than $5.2 billion. That same year, some 51 million Americans had their pharmaceutical benefits managed by Medco.

"INSTANT SUCCESS"

In his first annual report to stockholders following passage of Hatch-Waxman, Ed Pratt, the intense, fast-talking head of Pfizer, had only one word for the regulatory and competitive challenges facing his company. That word was "severe." It was an unusually ominous sentiment for someone like Pratt, a gregarious, go-ahead type who, by 1984, had captained the company for more than a decade and brought it to worldwide prominence.

Pratt was the latest incarnation of what was called the "Pfizer type." The originator of that type — and the man whose legacy shaped executives like Pratt — was a man named John McKeen. McKeen had died in 1978, but nevertheless loomed large over the company because it was he who, in the years after the Second World War, transformed Pfizer from a maker of refined chemicals (with which other companies made drugs) into a world-class manufacturer and marketer of its own drugs, mainly antibiotics. McKeen emphasized speed, innovation, and a ton of marketing savvy. As *Business Week* would later laud him, under John McKeen "the company displayed a kind of promotional hoopla more commonly identified with political and fraternal gatherings."

In real life, McKeen had also given to Pfizer its other main attributes: regulatory moxie and political pugnacity. This he demonstrated, in 1959, on a national stage in front of a national audience. The occasion was Senator Estes Kefauver's hearings into monopolistic pricing practices. True to form, when Kefauver got going on pharmaceuticals, the hearing took a dramatic turn. Kefauver accused Pfizer of withholding key safety data about its new diabetes drug, Diabenese, prompting a wave of negative headlines. But McKeen, who had been summoned to testify, noticed that there was a method to Kefauver's maddening media tactics. The senator always brought out his most weighty experts just before deadline, when reporters had to file their daily stories, resulting in the most incendiary charges making headlines and going unchallenged. McKeen, furious, decided to hit back, and set up his own "response center" of documents and press releases in the back of the Senate hearing room. As an internal Pfizer history notes: "When Senator Kefauver attempted to grab a headline out of sensational charges, Mr. McKeen rose from the audience and demanded that other doctors be permitted to respond immediately — on the spot. The doctors testified, and the resulting news reports carried — some even featured — Pfizer's response. Senator Kefauver had met his match in John McKeen."

Ed Pratt had been so impressed with that story that he commissioned a corporate history to preserve it in managerial agar and had it distributed to all of his top executives. The point: Among U.S. pharmaceuticals firms, Pfizer was different. It thought on its feet and, when necessary, went into the ring with its gloves off.

By the time of the negotiations over Hatch-Waxman, Pratt had also succeeded in the regulatory arena. He developed such a crack political team — its chief was an engaging Vietnam War hero named Steve Conafay — that he was able to convince even Henry Waxman to make an exemption for his new antiarthritic drug, Feldene. (Many referred to that subsection of Hatch-Waxman as "the Feldene amendment," something Waxman had to grin and bear and something over which Ed Pratt simply grinned.) That same year Pfizer worldwide sales approached $4 billion, with profits exceeding $500 million for the first time in the company's history.

Yet . . . "severe," the word that began the 1984 annual report, did not sound like the Ed Pratt of Pfizer's headiest days, did it?

But Pratt now knew that, with Hatch-Waxman, the old Pfizer ways — that of aggressive physician detailing to get new drugs established and the use of lobbying to keep generic competitors at bay — were no longer enough. If Pfizer was to survive, it would have to do a lot more, a lot faster. And that meant making big changes in management — in the core values of how the company was run.

No one knew this better than the enterprising folks in Pfizer's marketing department. For years, they had been stymied in the one arena in which they felt they could exert a particularly stimulating hand. That arena was research and development. Although Gerald Laubach, the head of the labs, had long championed teamwork in product development, he had specifically left out the marketers. They had no say in what was chosen as a promising chemical to develop and submit to the FDA for approval. Part of Laubach's resistance was political — the "head scientist" could not expect allegiance from his idealistic minions if they perceived him as a cave-in to the money guys. Part was purely managerial — Laubach's team process was already unwieldy enough, balancing many diverse departments. There was, of course, a new generation of more career-oriented scientists who were not against the idea of increasing productivity. But there was no leadership at the top for them. "There would be these very angry meetings, the twain-shall-never-meet science types versus the marketers," recalls Steve Conafay, who was present for many such confrontations. "The scientists thought that it should be science for science's sake and the salesmen were saying, 'Give me something to sell!'"

Then, in 1985, Pratt named a new head to Pfizer's prescription drug division, William C. Steere, Jr. Unlike his predecessor, Steere had no medical or scientific background, but rather he was a sales and marketing specialist. He had joined Pfizer in 1959 as a detail man. The son of William C. Steere, Sr., one of the twentieth century's most noted botanists, the younger Steere had never been engaged by the elder's scientific — or, for that matter, scholarly — inclinations. He had been a lackluster student at Stanford, mostly unnoticed by his peers. Back then, his mother recalled, he had been a "rather unfocused young man," but once young Bill understood "that he had to get on with a career" he "focused like a laser." At Pfizer, he had done just that, emerging as a brilliant salesman and marketing tactician. True, he could be maddeningly shy at times, and he hated foreign postings, required for anyone serious about climbing the pole to upper management, but by the time Bill Steere's name came to Ed Pratt's attention, there was no doubt who should become head of the pharmaceuticals division.

Steere arrived at the helm of the division just when Pratt and a number of senior scientists were coming to a hard conclusion: the old church-and-state divisions between marketing and R&D were no longer justified. John Niblack, then the vice president of medicinal products research, recalled that "marketing had certain ideas about what it wanted, how it wanted a product developed, and what attributes and features it wanted highlighted in a development program."

Steere vigorously championed a possible solution. The company would create two new kinds of management teams around every new drug, an Early Candidate Management Team and an Advanced Candidate Management Team. The former would include representatives from research, marketing, and sales. When a drug reached a stage when FDA submission looked likely, the first team would hand the portfolio over to the second, which was chaired by a marketing person. Both teams would report to a new central research division established by Steere. In the re-engineering-speak of the mid-1980s, when almost every large American company was rethinking how it did things, Steere was evangelical on the subject. "Our goal," he once explained, "was to communicate earlier on products to make sure that their development was such that when they entered the market, they'd be instant successes."

Instant successes! Dr. Barry Bloom, then the head of Pfizer research, recalls the sea change in Pfizer management and scientific circles as the Steere doctrine percolated downward. "For the first time we at R&D would have the insights of the commercial thinking that scientists often discounted or were oblivious of.

What we talked about were which indications an NDA [new drug application] should be filed for. The marketing and business people would, for the first time, have their say about what drugs would have the best shot on the market."

One of the first compounds to go through the process was fluconazole, or Diflucan, a powerful antifungal. The question before the committee was simple: Should the drug be developed at a high dose, which would make it effective for HIV patients, or at a low dose, for more common fungal infections. The former would be a difficult market, fraught with pricing issues; the latter would be more profitable. Steere liked to talk about how the company had taken the high road with Diflucan. "Neither side was willing to yield," he later wrote. "Finally, we formed a team of talented people from various areas of the company, giving them explicit instructions to bring an end to the standoff. We gave them no choice: we put them in a room and explained that nobody would leave until there was a plan that made sense for the whole company. In the end, the team designated the high-dosage approach."

If there was ever a drug candidate that could benefit from such synergy, it was one known around the company as sertraline, later branded as Zoloft. The compound had been kicked around by Pfizer scientists since the mid-1970s, when it emerged from research on antipsychotic molecules. Like Prozac and Paxil, Zoloft has certain properties that seemed to alleviate depression; the drug had some effect on serotonin levels — although, again like the others, no one could show just how that affected depression — and it was safer than the older antidepressants. You could not overdose on it. That said, there was, even to be charitable about it, a fudge factor in Zoloft. Like the other new antidepressants, it was no better at treating depression than older, "more dangerous" drugs, and patients — visions of Valium still trudging through their memory — were wary of taking a mood pill. Nevertheless, using the new candidate management committees, Steere pushed and prodded until Zoloft was ready for submission to the FDA.

By 1991, when Steere was named CEO of the entire company,

the candidate management system had succeeded in tearing down all the old walls. There was a new gusher of potential instant successes flowing from Pfizer labs to FDA reviewers. Steere was so elated that he moved Barry Bloom from R&D's traditional home base, in Groton, Connecticut, to an office down the hall from his at Pfizer's Manhattan headquarters. Then, in case no one had noticed, he called in Steve Conafay, then the head of political affairs, and issued a new managerial dictum. "He told me he had three priorities," recalls Conafay, who is now retired. "The first one was get marketing and research closer together. The second one was get marketing and research closer together. And then he said the third one was get marketing and research closer together." Everyone got the message.

And there would be no more perfect melding of message, man, and product than in Zoloft, which was approved by the FDA in December 1991. The new candidate committees, with their synergy and freewheeling discussions between scientists and marketing, produced a powerful new sales tool — one that might be called aspirational pill marketing. At the core of the new campaign was Zoloft's slogan "From depression, into the mainstream," in itself an odd choice because most depressed people were already in the mainstream, but never mind. With the slogan and a glut of samples went a steady stream of prescribing pads, notebooks, and freebies to physicians, all emblazoned with the same narrative tableau: a thirtyish supermom character in the process of performing all of the tasks expected of any upwardly mobile woman of the early 1990s. There was Zoloft Woman playing tennis (with a mean backhand), dancing with her husband, greeting her two children, giving a detailed financial presentation at work, walking with a friend, then jogging, then having dinner, presumably home-cooked, with hubby.

The Zoloft narrative was a not so subtle way to play to the newly emerging demographics of antidepressant use. Steere's marketing department knew, for example, that women were two to three times more likely than men to report that they were depressed, and that people under forty were three times more likely than their elders to report hopelessness and other symptoms. Of course, the Pfizer folks also knew that depression was a world-wide phenomenon, with many factors giving to its rise, among them the ascendance of individualism, the waning of belief systems, the erosion of the nuclear family and traditional sources of self-identification. Indeed, one study at the time indicated that many of the same elements of the Zoloft Woman campaign, with its unattainable ideal of beauty and grace combined with the perfect juggling of work and parenting, could also be one of the causes of depression in the first place. But that observation did not make it into the next iteration of the campaign.

Almost immediately, Steere knew he had a hit. Sales jumped. But how to take on Prozac, the real cash cow? Here was where Pfizer's medical affairs department, staffed with M.D.s and Ph.D.s, took over. As they saw it, the key was to hit Prozac in the side effects, where it was suffering from a number of negative articles in the press. Pfizer commissioned a series of highly technical studies that emphasized the chemical differences between Zoloft and other SSRIs — that it was, for example, less likely to react with other compounds in the body, or that it had a "better half-life," or a "cleaner" metabolic breakdown. These features were technically true, but, like saying that two ounces of vodka was better for you than two ounces of rum, they meant almost nothing the morning after. As David Healy, the British epidemiologist and expert on antidepressants, put it in his outstanding book *Let Them Eat Prozac*, "This marketing strategy produced lots of data — the appearance of science — but very few of these data were clinically relevant. It was immensely tedious, but it worked for Pfizer and Zoloft."

The new synergy was working in other ways as well. Steere's newly created central research division, engorged with marketing as well as scientific data, came up with a program, unimaginable in the old days, called CRAM, or Central Research Assists Marketing. For Zoloft, CRAM came up with two outreach programs, each one part-study, part–patient education. In one, dubbed "Prime M.D.," CRAM used its database to identify primary care physicians who might be open to educational programs about depression and Zoloft. These were, by and large, physicians with little or no training in psychiatry. But a little education, particularly in the managed care context, could go a long way toward making the untrained feel just confident enough to think they could diagnose depression. As Healy notes: "This of course made it likely that many of these doctors would go on to treat patients who had been identified as depressed, and that Zoloft would be the first drug tried."

The second CRAM program, dubbed "Rhythms," targeted the other end of the M.D. spectrum, focusing on leading academic clinicians. They were given millions to introduce their depressed clients to a series of Pfizer-created audio-visual presentations, to be viewed over the course of their treatment. The materials consisted of a twenty-eight-week series of newsletters and video-tapes, sent to patients' homes, about depression, why it was important to continue to take the drug even when they weren't sure it was working, why depression wasn't something to be ashamed of, and so on. A study of such patients, widely circulated by Pfizer in 1997, showed, unsurprisingly, that "a significantly higher percentage of patients in the Rhythms group said they were more satisfied with their treatment regimen than those who did not receive the program." It did not mention that almost any group of patients that gets more attention from their physicians — as was the case of all the Rhythms clients — do better than those who do not. (Such a phenomenon used to be called "doctoring.") Nor did the study deal with the troubling reality that Rhythms might also be encouraging patients to stay on a drug that might be harming them in unknown ways, say, via the complex suicide mechanism suspected in almost all the new antidepressants.

Central research, medical affairs, marketing — every department seemed to benefit from the new Steere synergy, but none more so than the sales department. Among the thousands of new recruits — Steere had ramped up hiring specifically for Zoloft — were many who instinctively understood the new Pfizer, and they had no trouble using the company's own technical materials in highly imaginative ways. Many began directly promoting the drug for premenstrual depression, using a new brochure via central research called "Reaching Out to Women." Others touted Zoloft for long-term use.

The problem was that all of these statements were either false, unsupported, misleading, or, worst of all, illegal. Steere's culture of synergy had become a culture so imbued with overreaching that even stock analysts from places like Smith Barney began saying, in the pages of the *New York Times*, no less, that Pfizer was "getting a little overaggressive." The FDA laid the blame squarely at the CEO's door. In September 1996, it took the unusual step of addressing one of its warning letters directly to Steere, instead of to the head of Pfizer regulatory affairs, as it usually did in such cases. In it, the agency directed Steere to "immediately cease" the dissemination of all unsupported claims and mandated that "within 15 days of the date of this letter, disseminate a message to all Pfizer sales representatives and marketing personnel involved in marketing and sales of Zoloft, instructing them to immediately cease" all unfounded claims for the drug. The agency also directed Steere to publish the message via paid advertisements in medical journals. This Steere did, with great umbrage, but only after a protracted and costly legal battle with the agency.

Meanwhile, sales of Zoloft neared the $2 billion mark, and Pfizer rose through the pharma ranks, from number fourteen in sales when Steere took charge in 1991 to number four in 1998. His research division continued to hatch new drugs. Among them were Norvasc, for hypertension, and Trovan, an antibiotic. Using the advanced candidate system, Steere relaunched Diflucan, originally developed for HIV infections, as a treatment for toenail fungus, at a low dose, but not a low price — it sold for $10 a hit. Sales were vigorous, but so was research and development spending. In fact, the bigger Pfizer got, the bigger were Steere's — and his board and chief stockholders' — aspirations. Size mattered. By 1998 Steere was saying that he would surpass Merck in sales by 2002.

Though many pressured him to purchase a pharmaceuticals benefit manager, as had Merck, Steere resisted. To those who pressed him, he liked to say, "We already have many ways of

drilling down to patients." To those who encouraged a merger —
and to those who circulated rumors that he was considering one
— he issued blunt denials that such had "no basis in fact." He
was truculent on the subject, though his immediate subordi-
nates, among them an up-and-coming vice president named
Hank McKinnell, quietly thought otherwise.

Then came Viagra, or sildenafil citrate, a compound originally
tested for treatment of angina. Although it proved a poor re-
liever of chest pain, Pfizer researchers early on noticed a remarkable side effect — it caused erections. Steere put the compound
through the screening process to come up with a marketable
drug; in other words, he asked research to "find" a "disease" that
regarded an erection as a "cure." The answer was a condition
dubbed "erectile dysfunction," or ED. Again, the in-house synergy worked brilliantly. Steere's medical affairs division funded
studies on ED and underwrote seminars on the subject. His sales
reps were tutored on the biology of smooth muscle tissue, the
physiological target of Viagra. "Viagra crystallized some things
I'd been thinking about," Steere told *Fortune* at the time. "It
struck me that a quality-of-life drug for aging would be a real
winner. Look at the volume in cosmetics, which are basically
nostrums that really don't do anything." In Viagra, Steere was
lucky: it had few true side effects, and those could be controlled
with a modicum of doctoring, unlike Zoloft.

Viagra, coming as it did after the FDA relaxed its rules on
DTC, was not only a commercial success, but also a veritable
cultural revolution in a pill, unleashing a new freedom in prescription drug advertising. Viagra became the Super Bowl drug,
the NFL drug, Bob Dole's drug. It ushered in the era of Internet
drug marketing. Among many other things it changed the billion-dollar porn industry, which changed Internet entertainment marketing. It did not exactly transform aging, as Steere had
hoped, but it did change youth. Viagra's presence was so huge, its
medical legitimacy established so quickly and so pithily, that
teenagers in Brooklyn were popping "V," as they called it, with
their "X," although why these kids needed help getting a boner
was not something anyone ever explored in the R&D depart-

ment. Viagra was safe, it was effective (as long as you were aroused), and it was everywhere.

Viagra's impact on Pfizer was — and there are no words that do not also sound like puns — enormous. First-year sales were $400 million, an unheard-of figure. In the United States alone, physicians were writing 275,000 prescriptions for it a week. By 2000, the worldwide sales figure was $1.5 billion. Even better, many large investors regarded the company as the best in the S&P 500. *Money* magazine readers and their proxies in the mutual funds business took note. Other pharma CEOs were expected to perform as well — or hit the road. Working out in the fitness center of Pfizer's Manhattan headquarters, Bill Steere was a happy man — the millennial embodiment of John McKeen.

And yet . . . Merck was still number one, and, Viagra jokes aside, by 2000, size in big pharma mattered. In investment circles, the talk centered on "market dominance" — a company could justify huge new investments in R&D only if it could somehow guarantee monopoly-like sales presence. In this way did discussions of pharmaceutical firms become like discussions of Hollywood movies. It was all about market presence. And, try as Bill Steere might, he could no longer force Pfizer's growth from within. For more instant successes, he would have to go shopping.

The company he would eventually buy would not only make Pfizer number one, but it would forever change the way the world did business with Pfizer, for better and for worse.

"WHY NOT LET THEM GET RICH?"

"Be pioneering!" Those were the words Joe Smith, the new head of Parke-Davis, liked to throw around in the early 1990s, and no wonder: Parke-Davis needed to find *something* good to sell. The previous decade had been a bust. The company had missed filing deadlines for potential blockbusters, and its R&D department had not passed regulatory muster with a series of other drugs. Wall Street analysts had already downgraded the stock. When Prudential Bache said the company had "a serious problem," all the "be pioneering" stuff suddenly started sounding like the whistling of a little boy walking down a long, dark alley. Smith grew frustrated. Hmm. The stockholders wanted a goddamn blockbuster; all he had was *be pioneering.*

Yet Smith's way had a lot more going for it than a first reading might suggest. Sure, the main thrust of his mission statement concerned discovering new drugs, but it also conjured another dynamic — that of being down for the count. With that threat, all kinds of never-before-uttered plans and ideas bubbled up. Call it the comet-is-going-to-hit-the-earth school of motivational theory.

One new idea came to Smith from an outside marketing consultant, Richard Vanderveer. Vanderveer was a Temple University–trained psychologist who had become interested in social research — how and why groups of people make decisions — before launching a career in medical marketing. Articulate, razor-sharp in the analytical skills department, Vanderveer spent much of his commercially formative years at a company called Intercontinental Marketing Service. IMS was the original pharmaceutical marketing firm; its main product is a huge database of information on prescription drug sales, which it purchased from individual pharmacies and then used to tailor advertising and marketing campaigns for drug makers. The patient information was anonymous, but the data gave marketers a good idea of which prescription drugs were selling, what geographical areas were slow to adopt new ones and which were fast, whether prescriptions were being refilled, and so forth. But there was no data about individual physicians and their prescribing behavior.

Vanderveer learned the IMS system and then went on to work at Medco, the huge prescription mail-order house that Merck acquired in 1992. Medco had the physician data — who prescribed what, when, and how. Vanderveer saw tremendous potential in a marriage of the IMS and Medco databases, which is exactly what happened when Medco and IMS came to an understanding to share the data not long after the Merck-Medco deal. When that occurred, Vanderveer went to Parke-Davis and Joe Smith with a vision. Smith gave him fifteen minutes to paint the picture. "I told Joe that he needed to institute a micromarketing program," Vanderveer recalls. "I told him the company needed to target individual physicians with tailored information that we knew would resound with them as individuals, instead of carpet-bombing them all with the same data." Smith bought in and funded a trial micromarketing program.

The trial involved a relatively new Parke-Davis drug, Loestrin, a low-estrogen birth control pill. Using the new IMS-Medco data, Vanderveer answered a number of questions about how to market the drug effectively: Which physicians were already high prescribers of birth control pills? Who, among them, was already overly committed to competitors like Ortho? Knowing that would tell Parke-Davis not to waste marketing dollars on that physician. Most importantly, since Loestrin's niche was women who were afraid of higher-dose estrogen tablets: Which physicians were writing low-dose prescriptions of existing drugs? Then, among those patients, how often did they let their prescription lapse, thus indicating displeasure with the current low dose? Now plug in the more affluent Zip Codes of Washington, D.C., say. Blink: There was your target. Now you had the names of all physicians treating women frustrated with existing low-dose meds who also, because of their Zip Code, were likely to be upper-middle- to upper-class and well educated. Bingo: The result of these parameters, says Vanderveer, was that "the data put the detail person in a simpatico headset with the doctor." The system could then use Merck's extensive biographical information on thousands of physicians — where they lived, went to school, etc. — to help them put an extra personal point on the sales call. To further that, the Loestrin sales group was recruited from among the company's ob/gyn sales reps, many of whom were former ob/gyn nurses who could talk knowledgeably and intimately about the benefits of a lower-dose pill. The carpet-bombers' tactic had morphed into the pharmaceutical equivalent of a cozy tea party for pills.

The results of the campaign were strong — not overwhelming, but strong enough for Joe Smith to encourage the micromarketing approach across the company. As Vanderveer recalls, "He was a happy executive."

But happiness remained a fleeting experience in the Parke-Davis executive suite. Warner-Lambert, the parent company, continued to flail; it was indicted for, and eventually pled guilty to, criminal charges for faulty manufacturing. Earnings remained crummy. Smith was discharged upward, to pioneer a different division. By 1995, reports of a takeover were rampant. There seemed no way to save the company.

Yet something different *had* happened. Micromarketing *had* pointed a new way. Getting into the "simpatico headset" of physicians by using data *had* worked. The company just needed to find the right drug on which to use Vanderveer's new tools, and the right executive to use them.

Anthony Wild, the man Warner-Lambert finally hired to save the company, arrived with the perfect amalgam of talents. He was trained in physical chemistry but had spent almost his entire career on the business side of the pharmaceuticals industry. Much of that had been spent in various foreign operations for Schering-Plough. In Japan, he had spearheaded a number of that company's new drug rollouts, among them the popular allergy pill Claritin. He was charming, engaged, genuinely optimistic, and agile. In short, everything the board — and stockholders — would want in a leader.

Wild had also been around long enough to know that taking a new job with an old-line pharmaceuticals firm, regardless of its storied past, carried huge potential for career destruction. When Warner-Lambert recruiters came calling, he went right to the sore spot: Wasn't the company in trouble? Yes, they admitted, the company had fallen on hard times. But there was a possible boon in the making. The Parke-Davis division anticipated the approval of two new drugs, one for high cholesterol called Lipitor, one for type 2 diabetes, called Rezulin. Both drugs had huge market potential, and the executive who presided over their successful launch would flourish, both professionally and personally. Was he up to the challenge?

Wild was. But he also knew a lot about the internal politics of Warner-Lambert, how the conglomerate often sabotaged and beggared the drug division's ability to exploit new drugs. So he presented his recruiters with his survival plan for the company, and for himself. There were, he said, a couple of existing Parke-Davis drugs that seemed undersold, among them Neurontin, which was approved for treatment of epilepsy, along with Loestrin and an antihypertensive named Accupril. Here was his proposal: If he could raise the sales of these drugs to 15 percent of their respective markets, he said, would Warner-Lambert guarantee that he, as head of Parke-Davis, could use those profits to promote Lipitor and Rezulin when they were approved? A deal was struck.

Even before he landed in the United States, Wild was hammering away at creating a new Parke-Davis culture. The first problem was the gloom and doom, he said. That inhibited creativity. "The low-risk approach can end up as the high-risk approach," he explained in a later interview. "You can do nothing until you die, which is what was happening at Parke-Davis — everything was about cutting costs, then getting fewer results, then getting more cost cutting." An example: When he asked why Loestrin wasn't growing faster, the reply was that "the sales force is too small." He then faxed the people who would be his top management team, asking them to fax him back a list of things they thought he should do in his first ninety days — things that would "incentivize" sales. Unsurprisingly, many of the suggestions boiled down to pay raises for sales reps — and Parke-Davis did not have the money for that. "We decided to hold a national sales conference" to come up with a way.

Sales representatives in most large companies are paid in a complex system of advances, quotas, year-end bonuses, and incentives. At Parke-Davis, incentives — essentially extra pay for hitting quarterly goals — were limited by a rigid system of internal caps. Caps were a way to keep the incentive payments from getting out of hand and eating into overall profits. But that policy obviously took the steam out of the company's younger, hungrier reps, the very people who could help sales the most. That was wrong, Wild decided. At the sales meeting, held in San Francisco, he uttered the previously unutterable: "Why are all these caps here?"

"Because you can't have people making endless incentives," came the response from the company's older hands.

"I said, 'Why?' Why not let them get rich?"

As Wild recalls: "We announced we were taking off the caps, and the sales force went nuts! The San Francisco meeting was like a huge black cloud being blown away finally. I told them: 'Believe in yourselves!'"

As it turned out, the biggest believers were those charged with increasing sales of Neurontin, for years a reliable but modest performer in the company's anti-epilepsy cabinet. This was because Neurontin was approved only for adjuvant therapy, for people suffering from seizures that were not well controlled by conventional seizure medications. That made its market small. It was approved only in relatively low doses, further shrinking its potential. Its side effects seemed relatively benign. The drug — its chemical name was gabapentin — was also intriguing to a number of people in the sales department. For years they had been hearing a small but steady number of comments from some doctors who had experimented with the drug off label, using it to treat neuropathic pain, bipolar disorder, attention deficit disorder, as monotherapy for seizures (instead of as an adjuvant) — even for migraine, restless leg syndrome, and alcohol and drug withdrawal. Yet there was no reliable evidence proving Neurontin's benefits in treating these conditions. It was all anecdotal. Trials to establish such claims — the kind needed for a new drug application — were expensive, and there was still a huge chance that they would fail. And because Neurontin was coming off patent in just four years anyway, why bother with such expensive trials? For the newly revved-up sales department, Neurontin was like having a bag of Halloween candy that was stapled shut. The question was: How could they increase its sales without overtly promoting its off-label use, which was illegal?

The answer came from a Parke-Davis division known as medical liaisons. Medical liaisons are a drug company's backup team. They are usually M.D.s or Ph.D.s, with deep understandings of the gray areas of any given drug's uses. They read the tiny case study summaries appearing in offbeat medical journals, stay abreast of big clinical trials, and study the reports coming through physicians using the company's own drugs, reports that can be, by turns, encouraging, alarming, or, usually, frustrating.

Clear causality between a drug and a benefit is a difficult thing to fathom, and medical liaisons know this in spades.

The main use of a medical liaison, from the point of view of a sales rep, is as a distributor of off-label information. Sales reps cannot do that — such is considered illegal promotion of an un-approved use. But they can get such information to an experi-mentally inclined customer-physician via the liaison, as long as the physician initiates the request for contact. These rules may seem to the outsider like the elaborate posturing of a Kabuki per-formance, but they are the framework that keeps — or used to keep — a bunch of twenty-three-year-old sales reps from run-ning around and making up new uses for powerful drugs with only a scintilla of evidence. Liaisons, and the departments that supported them, thus performed a moderating influence on sales, occasionally useful but more often like a parental scold. The question to Parke-Davis's Neurontin team was: How can we incentivize our medical affairs guys, who could then incentivize all those off-label-writing physicians? The stakes were huge, af-ter all, with the market for pain meds alone reaching well into the nine-figure range.

One answer was breathtakingly simple: start recruiting medi-cal liaisons not from the ranks of M.D.s and Ph.D.s, but from the ranks of . . . sales reps, which is exactly what Parke-Davis began to do. According to a number of depositions and thousands of pages of internal company documents, that single change quickly altered its entire medical liaison department. Dr. David Franklin, one of the few non-salespeople to be hired at the time as a medical liaison, described the transformative effects:

At Parke-Davis, many of the medical liaisons were hired directly out of the sales department. They were all trained in sales tech-niques, and compensated, in part, on the basis of sales. They had no discernable scientific or medical functions. They had no com-munication or interaction with Parke-Davis['s] actual medical research divisions. The medical liaisons were assigned to act as teams with the regular sales representatives. They were given lists of doctors for "cold calls," based on the size of the doctors' prac-tices and their ability to prescribe Neurontin. They were provided with a package of monetary incentives to offer to physicians to get involved in the Parke-Davis programs.

The scale and the breadth of the change were stunning, both in terms of the sales potential and legal downside. In Tony Wild's newly energized Parke-Davis culture, however, the task was not to scale down but to find ways to ramp up. One way was to educate the liaisons about the law. In April 1996, a former FDA official and a company lawyer held a mandatory liaison seminar on the subject. The first part was videotaped. The pair began by saying that "if you get caught violating the FDA rules, you're on your own and acting without the company's knowledge or permission." They then went on to say that "you must have a physician information request form (IRF) for each call, you must provide fair and balanced presentation, you can't close or sell, you can't promote a drug off label, you can't promote a drug preapproval, you must keep accurate records of your activities, [and] you can't solicit an inquiry."

The video camera was then turned off. What followed was a very different, "candid" presentation of what Parke-Davis expected: "We expect you to do your job out there and stay focused on sales. Don't worry about this." Then the lawyer and the former FDA official restated their original presentation in more pragmatic terms: "If you're cold-calling with a sales representative, have him fill out the IRF form, so you are covered. You're not out there to help the [competitors], and the doctors know it, so don't worry about being balanced. Look, without sales there is no Parke-Davis. We all have to sell on some level. Be careful about this, but everyone wants to know about atorvastatin [Lipitor, not yet approved]. Just don't leave anything behind. Above all, don't put anything in writing."

Slowly but surely, the liaisons became a seamless part of the sales and marketing departments. They went to the same meetings, heard the same pep talks, were promised the same incentives. In one meeting they were promised an all-expenses-paid cruise to the Bahamas if the company hit certain sales goals for Neurontin and Accupril. "The only way we will make it [to the

Bahamas] is if you as a group take ownership of the task and get out there and aggressively move share," one speaker from the marketing department proclaimed.

> You have to be aggressive . . . don't take no for an answer. If the rep doesn't close, you close. If the rep is seeing the wrong docs, you see the right ones. If a high-decile [high-prescribing] practice isn't using Neurontin, get in there, do your thing, then ask why. Tell them that if their patients aren't on Accupril, they're doing them a disservice. Tell them the endothelial dysfunction story [the disease process that is Accupril's target], about the reversal of CAD [coronary artery disease], everything, I don't care, but you're wasting your time and our money if you don't ask for the new script [order] when you're through . . .

The new, pragmatic force of liaisons soon dominated the Neurontin team. The result was explosive: Not only were more and more physicians, particularly those whose IMS-Medco data showed that they were "high writers" for pain and bipolar disorder, hearing about Neurontin, but they were writing new prescriptions! Sales figures moved up. Just as remarkable was the wave of innovation coming out of the liaisons themselves. Much of their work, once almost entirely focused on carefully discerning the truth of new scientific data, now centered on ways to further educate, engage, and involve high-writing physicians. In other words, to incentivize them and make them part of the Neurontin family.

One way was to give them 100 milligrams of money. Although it is illegal for a drug company to pay physicians to prescribe a drug, it is not illegal, technically, to pay them for being special consultants. Parke-Davis paid thousands of physicians to become such consultants; the only (rarely enforced) requirement was to attend one meeting. Almost all of the money went to doctors who "wrote" Neurontin heavily, particularly those for bipolar and pain. Then there was the so-called preceptor program, in which physicians were paid $350 every time they allowed a Parke-Davis rep to visit. The visits almost always included discussions of patients and often resulted in sales reps meeting actual patients. In one case, documented in internal company papers, a sales rep was able not only to meet with patients, but to then convince the physician to write off-label prescriptions to treat the patients.

There was more. The company established a Parke-Davis Speakers Bureau, paying high-writing Neurontin "thought leaders" to go out and spread the word. There was, of course, no solid data in the form of clinical trials, but there was data generated from less strict studies. These were called "case studies," and they, too, were paid for by the company. Usually they consisted of loose observations by Speakers Bureau physicians, who had been paid on a case-by-case basis to write up each patient history and response to Neurontin. It was the kind of daisy-chain enterprise that made mainstream experts in clinical trials shudder, as it was conducted without even the most rudimentary of scientific guidelines.

And, as in any marketing-driven enterprise, once the gray areas are banished, color emerges, first at the edges, then at the red-hot center. By April 1996, blatant off-label promotion had become the standard. At a recorded meeting of marketing managers that month, the Parke-Davis executive John Ford stated the company's expectations:

"I want you out there every day selling Neurontin. Look, this isn't just me, it's come down from Morris Plains [headquarters] that Neurontin is more profitable than Accupril so we need to focus on Neurontin . . . We all know that Neurontin's not growing for adjunctive therapy [its approved indication]. Besides that's not where the money is. Pain management, now that's money. Monotherapy, that's money.

"We don't want to share these patients with everybody, we want them on Neurontin only. We want their whole drug budget, not a quarter, not a half, the whole thing . . . we can't wait for them to ask, we need to get out there and tell them out front. Dinner programs, CME [continuing medical education] programs, consultantships, all work great, but don't forget the one-on-one. That's where we need to be, holding their hand and whispering in their ear, Neurontin for pain, Neurontin for monotherapy, Neurontin for bipolar, Neurontin for everything . . . I don't want to see a single patient coming off Neurontin before they've been up to at least 4,800 milligrams a day.

"I don't want to hear that safety crap either — every one of you should take one just to see there is nothing. It's a great drug."

"Gloom and doom," one might safely say, were things of the past at Tony Wild's Parke-Davis.

Sales exploded. Wild put more programs in place to encourage the "new enterprise culture." And by now, the new drugs — drugs that he was promised a big budget to promote — were nearing readiness.

The new drugs: they could ensure that the company would not only survive, but dominate. Both Lipitor and Rezulin targeted huge new growth markets, those with high cholesterol and those with type 2 diabetes. In many ways, both drugs were products of the newly loosened and speeded-up regulatory processes that the industry had been engineering since Hatch-Waxman. Both had benefited in their development from research and researchers from the NIH, who had been freed from old conflict-of-interest limits by the Engman-era Bayh-Dole Act. Both benefited from that same era's recommendations that only one or two studies should suffice for approval. And both drugs benefited from the regulatory speeding up that happened when patient groups got involved in drug approvals, courtesy of Gerry Mossinghoff, as well as from the Prescription Drug User Fee Act, which put economic pressure on the FDA to hasten approvals, particularly for drugs that treated novel conditions.

By 1996, indeed, agile executives like Wild understood that the approval process itself could be used to the company's advantage. If the stodgy world of medical liaisons could be revved up, his thinking went, so could the equally old-world ways of regulatory affairs — the people entrusted with making the company's scientific and medical case for FDA approval. There were new ways to get a drug on the market faster. One of these was known as "expedited review." The FDA grants an expedited review when a company can show that a new drug treats a condition that other drugs don't. As Wild tells it, with Lipitor "we had a very clever regulatory crew who figured out that we could file for familial hypercholesterolemia, which is a very small group of patients in the United States. We used some South African data, because there it is a genetic thing. We included that data in the label, and we got approval in five months!" The same tack worked with Rezulin. Rather than simply applying as a me-too drug for treatment of type 2 diabetes, Parke-Davis emphasized that the drug was needed for people who wanted to take fewer insulin shots.

There was something else going on in regulatory affairs. In the FDA advisory committee meeting for Rezulin, for example, company reps presented unclear safety data about liver complications, then promised to submit clarifying data if the drug was approved. It was, but they didn't. For reasons never completely explained, the FDA accepted the promise for future data and then signed off on Rezulin. The open window had become a gaping hole. Wild had his second potential blockbuster.

With the approvals, Wild grew convinced that a new era was at hand for Parke-Davis. Especially with Lipitor. "When I arrived, the sales forecast for Lipitor was three quarters of a million in annual sales by the fourth year," he recalls. "It was perceived as being difficult to carve out a new niche, as there were so many other statins. I dove into the data and became convinced that it was a much bigger product. We called a meeting and everyone was quite excited. I threw out a thought: This product is good enough for a twenty-five percent share. People fell off their chairs: no way! It was scary to think about being that big." But to be that big, Parke-Davis would need a marketing partner — a bigger company with the sales and distribution network that long-impoverished Parke-Davis lacked. That meant that the company would have to give up a percentage of Lipitor profits in exchange. After a long and furious battle with Warner's chairman, who did not want to give up anything in the launch of the company's first new product in a decade, Wild prevailed. The company they picked, Bill Steere's booming Pfizer, was a perfect fit: it had no competing product and it had a huge sales force of aggressive, young detail people.

Once the drug was approved and a partner picked, Wild pushed the marketing division to go back to the IMS-Medco data to come up with a way to get close, this time not just with physicians but also with patients. The man he picked to head the new direct-to-consumer campaign, Robert Ehrlich, was something of a departure from the usual pharma recruit. Ehrlich hailed from Parke-Davis's consumer goods division in Tokyo, where he was in charge of everything, as he said, "from gum to Tums." Reading over the Lipitor label, then looking at studies of consumer awareness, he had a revelation: the campaign shouldn't even mention such bummers as heart attacks and cardiovascular disease, the reasons for the drug's existence. Instead the campaign should be . . . fun. "We had a fairly good efficacy advantage, and a statin was by then well understood by doctors and patients," he recalls. "So we didn't feel that we had to discuss heart attacks. That would have been a confusing message.

"Instead, we took a consumer insight: people liked to compare their cholesterol numbers! They don't like to talk in terms of 'I prevented a heart attack.' We did not think that they cared about studies. They liked to talk about their numbers." That was what the ads would emphasize; two guys, or two gals, comparing their "scores." To design the ads, Ehrlich picked Bates Advertising. Bates was legendary in consumer goods campaigns. The agency's principals, Bob Frohlich and Bob Tabor, were credited with coming up with such lines as "Certs: It's two-two-two mints in one!" and "Rolaids spells relief." Their Lipitor campaign debuted during the hit TV show *ER* in February 1998, only months after FDA approval.

The sales response was nothing short of revolutionary. The combination of DTC, physician detailing, and the sheer muscle of Bill Steere's sales force pushed the drug to the top of the statin charts.

Next came Rezulin. Rezulin was a different matter. It was the first in a new class of drugs, known as glitazones. It did not necessarily work better than other drugs that treated type 2 diabetes, but it did have advantages: Rezulin might allow a type 2 patient who was taking insulin (and many did) as part of treatment to reduce his number of daily injections. But physicians did not really care about that. They mainly cared about whether the drug improved control of blood sugar, which Rezulin did, but not to the extent that might warrant a switch. Patients, on the other hand, cared deeply about their daily number of shots, regardless of how well their blood sugar was controlled. "There was a missing discussion — that was the challenge — how to stimulate that discussion between patient and physician," recalls Ehrlich. Only with that discussion would Rezulin sales take off.

Stimulating the discussion was done through Parke-Davis's sophisticated new detailing methods; IMS-Medco data could pinpoint which physicians used which drugs for type 2. Medical journal ads were taken out emphasizing "better control" of blood sugar. The same kind of paid preceptorships used so effectively with a relatively benign drug like Neurontin were now employed for Rezulin; high-writing diabetes doctors were paid to accept sales calls on Rezulin and to share the data of patients who might benefit from the drug. To the consumer, the message was different. "To the consumer, it was 'I can reduce my shots,'" recalls Ehrlich. "That was the wow factor for patients." The campaign also focused heavily on the emerging type 2 diabetes epidemic in the nation's Latino communities, with ads in Spanish. The side effects information on the other side was in English.

Within months of its launch, Rezulin had racked up $250 million in sales. Like Lipitor, it seemed destined for blockbuster status. Wild was promoted to executive vice president of his parent company, Warner-Lambert.

There was, in all of this, the usual carping of the spoilsports, the non–team players, the inflexible guys who still thought in terms of win-lose rather than win-win. In the case of Neurontin, there were a few medical liaisons who felt that the off-label action that Wild had instigated was nothing short of "brazen criminal behavior," as one put it. They were ignored or sidelined, politely. Similar issues emerged with Rezulin: Why was the safety information for Latinos left in English? What was that about?

Yet in the new, incentivized pharma era, when every department from R&D to regulatory affairs had a greater, grander vision of what was possible, such fretting was easily dismissed, or shunted off to some dismal cubicle in some New Jersey regional office. Almost without exception, the industry viewed Parke-Davis and Wild as the pivotal figures in the most remarkable turnaround in recent pharma history.

In 2000, Bill Steere just had to buy the company — and everything that came with it. By then, with almost all major players resorting to mergers to boost market ascendancy, U.S. companies were the dominant force in the worldwide pharmaceutical industry. In one generation, they had been unbound, ungagged, retooled, and, finally, recast as the leading edge of the national economy.

Only slowly would Americans awaken to what that might mean in their daily lives, in what was happening all around them . . .

We Love It!

How the New Pharma Used Its New Muscle to Create a New . . . You

IF, IN THE 1990s, Dr. David Kessler had struck fear into the hearts of those who wanted to market drugs in the new synergistic way — either via DTC or off label — by 2002 he was, strangely at least to outsiders, suddenly acquiescent. "I was wrong about DTC," Kessler would easily admit to those who asked him about his one-time bane. Then he cited the facts: every time he looked at a study of DTC, the benefits outweighed the downside, the side he had so worried about when he was head of the FDA.

To the skeptic, Kessler, now the nattily clad dean of Yale Medical School, would proffer opinion polls and consumer surveys. Citing a study by the Kaiser Family Foundation, he noted that consumers who had viewed DTC ads were more aware of disease treatment options than those who hadn't seen the ads. That, he thought, was a plus. Patients with high cholesterol and asthma who'd seen DTC ads were more likely to be aware of new drugs for those conditions than were those who hadn't viewed the spots. Ditto, yes? DTC ad viewers were also much more aware of a given drug's side effects than nonviewers. Who could argue with that? True, the Kaiser study showed the commercial bonus as well: 30 percent of DTC viewers go to their physicians in response to an ad, and 44 percent get a prescription for the advertised product. But Kessler did not say much about that.

No, Americans — doctors, patients, insurers — loved DTC, Kessler concluded. Yes, there was the endless carping by a narrow group of regulatory stalwarts, and yes, DTC could be made better and more helpful, no doubt. But in general, as he declaimed to the DTC National Conference in April 2002, he, David Kessler, the late twentieth century's most activist FDA chief, had been wrong about prescription drug advertising. Moreover, the assembled pharma execs — many of the same ones he'd vilified in the 1990s — could count on his continued support if they focused on the need to educate consumers about "the most serious conditions." As Kessler concluded, "The more you wear the public health hat, the more drugs you'll sell in the end." The audience at the DTC National clapped loudly.

The industry group Rx Insight, founded and run by Bob Ehrlich, Tony Wild's enterprising marketing director for Lipitor, put Kessler on the cover of its trade magazine, *DTC Perspectives*. It was a very simpatico moment.

By 2002, spending on DTC was soaring. And although more and more of the ads were sounding exactly like the ones once envisioned over twenty-five years ago by a fretting Justice Rehnquist ("Feeling Sad? Anxious? Tired?" was the new line for Zoloft), few could quibble with the success of a new industry in the making. By 2001 the investment in DTC prescription advertising had risen to $1.8 billion. That same year saw another important shift as well: drug companies spent more on ads in newspapers and magazines than they did in medical journals.

Yet it was not simply spending patterns that had changed. Pharma was now using its hard-won new freedoms to market pills as if they were any other consumer product, and with that came a mighty transformation in the way Americans use prescription drugs to run their lives.

UNCLE PHARMA, TRIBAL LEADER

The sheer mass of the DTC boom conjured huge, once unthinkable transformations. In the field of prescription drug marketing, there rose a vast new network of stars and institutions. Heads of marketing from traditional consumer goods firms began to migrate to big pharma, bringing with them a whole new set of tools. The guru of Pfizer's DTC efforts hailed from Kraft's cereal and yogurt division, and the new head of the company's Lipitor DTC program came via the Flintstones vitamin division of Bayer and the Softsoap division of Colgate. At Merck, the DTC guru came via Maxwell House coffee.

No single institution brought together the talent and the new ideas as did the Pharmaceutical Marketing Congress, known as the PMC, held every year in Philadelphia's Wyndham Franklin Hotel, just down the street from Jan Leschly's old haunt at SmithKline. The PMC is part idea mart, part technology confab, part networking conference. Think of it as the world's fair of pharmaceutical marketing, the place where the quest for a better pharma-consumer connection goes high-tech and high-touch.

The stars of the PMC universe are not traditional ones, although at breakfast or lunch one might see a celebrity give a keynote speech — former Wonder Woman Lynda Carter on the dangers of irritable bowel syndrome, or *Happy Days*'s Tom Bosley on mental health issues. Rather, they are people like Pat Kelly, the president of U.S. pharmaceuticals for Pfizer and, unquestionably, the definitive lead guitar player in the rocking world of modern drug marketing. Kelly cut his teeth at Pfizer after graduation from Duke and then rose through the ranks with hugely successful marketing efforts for Viagra, Lipitor, and Celebrex. He is an amiable, serious man, with a tiny bald spot amid a closely cropped head of curly hair. His cherubic countenance alone would make him highly trustworthy as your dentist.

In September 2002, despite his and the industry's success, Kelly painted a grim picture for the PMC audience listening to his keynote. Up on the giant ballroom screen at the Wyndham Franklin he flashed a huge picture of a woman as the target of a knife thrower to drive his points home. "Our markets, customers, and products are all under assault!" he proclaimed. The industry was being hit hard by generics, by pressure from HMOs and pharmaceuticals benefit managers to ratchet down prices, by advocacy groups that were constantly finking on pharma for over-the-top marketing practices, and from the media, particularly from the *Wall Street Journal* and Peter Jennings, who seemed to pump from a deep well of antipharma news stories that year. ("That gawd-dam Jennings," a woman sitting in front muttered in a gravelly whisper.)

Kelly then queued up another visual, this one the "I'm not gonna take it anymore" scene from the movie *Network*. "It's time to fight back!" Kelly said. But that didn't mean fighting with Peter Jennings or the *Journal*. In fact, he said, the problem wasn't those external factors at all; it was a matter of changing the way the industry thought about *itself* and its products. "We are challenged that our products are too high-priced, and we tend to respond with a rational answer to an emotional question," Kelly explained. "Now, doing *that* is at the core of what we do, but it's a way we must find our way *out* of." As Kelly saw it, there were three ways of branding products: the rational, show-and-tell model, based on science and free samples; the emotional-situational method, based on humor and human experience; and the spiritual-ethical method, based on attracting people to their better selves and the institutions aligned with such. Invoking Maslow's hierarchy of needs, Kelly threw down a challenge: pharma must move toward the emotional way of marketing, because "in that way we can move toward the spiritual-ethical method." And more: "We must find a way to market beyond just product."

Beyond product? By that, Kelly meant that pharma, like other giant industries, could no longer simply sell *things*. It had to sell lifestyle. And to do that, it had to transform the very core of the pharma-patient transaction. The whole notion of a hard sell by a company to a helpless patient had to be turned into one of a smart choice made by a continually empowered partner. "We have to figure out the modern patient's real needs," he said. "That will help us build a partnership out of a relationship. We have to get closer to the customer, connecting and exchanging information."

And the way to do that, he went on, was to support two interrelated things: patient compliance and patient persistence. The two issues were, as everyone in the Wyndham Franklin ballroom that day knew, key and often sore spots in the pharma CEO suite. Compliance and persistence referred to the fact that up to half of all patients either did not take their meds as directed (noncompliance with the doctor's orders) or did not take them for the often long periods of time required, as was the case with almost all of the industry's top-selling drugs for chronic disease (nonpersistence). Kelly summed up: "There are still a profound number of patients who don't know they should be our patients!"

What should they do? The industry needed to "pull" patients using the new information technologies, the media, and the Internet, all of which could drive people into the new relationship — the partnership — with pharma, Uncle Pharma, if you will. "We have to use that to push them into the camp of increased life expectancy," the ultimate lure, Kelly said. The "way in" was to make pharma into a kind of compliance and persistence counselor, one with deep pockets and the ability to "incent" patients, just as it did doctors, into Uncle Pharma's "camp."

The crowd roared. Kelly had found a way out of the encroaching morass. Pharma. Patient. Friends.

Apart from Kelly's allusions to pharma's "spiritual" closeness to patients, his ideas were already part and parcel of modern mainstream consumer marketing theory. In short, what he was talking about was consumer tribalism. By conjuring brand tribalism — an intense, interactive, and information-driven promotion of a product *and the values it is made to seem to embody* — a company can not only gain new customers, but also hold on to the old ones, which is crucial to long-term profitability. Think "rebel," "cool," "plush," "young," and think . . . Virgin Records and Virgin Airlines. Then go to the company's Web sites and get a free gift for signing up to be part of its "club," which will then give you automatic notices of new releases, discounts, upcoming concerts, special deals. Make these visits often enough, and soon the Virgin marketing people will be able to customize the promotions they send you, maximizing the potential for a sale and minimizing the hassle to you of unnecessary promos. Thus is created the Virgin tribe. That tribe then sustains personal identification with the product. It is a way for a product to become the focus of primal tribal impulses — of belonging, of shared belief, of language, taboo, and sanction.

The tribal connections for big pharma were obvious — disease, patients, pills. It was a natural. But the notion itself had always been uttered quietly in industry circles. It simply sounded too heavy-handed. Pharma. Tribes. It even scared the hell out of the marketing people. But as early as 1999, pharma's priciest consultants — the guys and gals who got five or, yes, six figures a day for their opinions — were talking tribe. In 1999, Patrick Dixon, a British futurist who, as one business magazine put it, "lives in the year 2010 and sees tomorrow as history," took up the subject. The occasion was a presentation to high-level managers at Glaxo. Projecting a list of the drug company's problems onto a giant video screen, Dixon then flashed another, contrasting slide. This one showed the Sara Lee brand of pastries next to a happy child. If pharma could somehow create the same visceral equation between consumers and its products, the future would not only be profitable, but less vulnerable. Dixon then sent up the Glaxo label and proclaimed: "All great drugs create tribes!" Finally someone had said it!

Back at the PMC, people were finally saying a lot of things. Consider Raymond Sacchetti, the head of "compliance and persistency" at Bristol-Myers Squibb. Sacchetti had made a study of patient compliance and what he called "adherence marketing," and he could *prove* that DTC resulted in better persistence. "If you do a hundred sixty days of DTC ads," he told the audience, "well, you get a thirty-five percent rate of compliance after twelve months. But if you do two hundred fifty days of DTC ads, you get sixty-five percent!" It could be a lot better, he said, if HMOs were not so chintzy in their reimbursement departments, constantly making bigger and bigger demands on everyone to justify long drug regimens. That's why increasingly motivated patients were critical to pharma's business. Yet these, he believed, would only come when patients trusted big pharma a lot more: "We want people to feel they can snuggle up to us at night." And that could happen only at "the magic moment."

What was the magic moment? It was when the first prescription was written. After all, "The doctor sits *in loco parentis*," Sacchetti explained. The first prescription was thus the most powerful moment — its clarity and drama determined whether a patient got motivated enough to comply and persist. Pharma, he said, needed to target more resources into sculpting that doctor's-office drama. There was another aha! moment.

The theme was then picked up by a number of other presenters. Brian Roberts, a pharma brand consultant, focused on the emerging database search tools in CRM, or customer retention management. Using data from hospitals and the American Medical Association, for example, one could analyze any given physician as part of a "physician needs cluster." Some were "aggressive science leaders." Others were "aggressive business managers." Some were "nonaggressive science leaders" but were "aggressive patient treaters." By using such data, Roberts said, "we can calculate the strategic value of each physician!" That would help individual pharma reps change the pitch to different physicians. A "physician who does not feel comfortable with a drug due to its side effects" would not get the same pitch as a doctor who was an "aggressive business manager."

What about marketing to women? Many believed such was the future grand lode, but not until pharma really understood women. As Gail Ludmeyer, the head of Wyeth's women's health initiative, explained, "Traditionally, women are seekers of information, but now they are barraged, and more confused than ever. We need to give their physicians information to un-confuse them." One way to do that was to recognize, as Pfizer's Ruth Merkatz said, that "women are logically emotional." Pfizer's localized marketing approach to the cardiovascular segment, she said, was having tremendous success with things like a recent "Heart Party," held in Boston just after a slew of high-profile cardiovascular and women's health studies were released. It was a logic and emotion party.

Public relations had to change as well. If you wanted to ensure that a lot of prescriptions for a new drug were written within the first ninety days of a drug's launch — the thumbnail test of success was now down to three months — you had to start doing public relations long before commencement of sales, about eighteen months before. Sander Flaum, a longtime pharma PR and marketing hand, outlined exactly what was working for his clients. "You have to pinpoint your early-adopting high writers and incent your sales reps to target them and them only," he said. Such high writers had an enormous influence on others in their profession, as well as on hospital formulary boards, which decide which new drugs to use. You also had to find well-spoken "thought leaders" and make sure that they were talking up the drug far in advance of its launch, or even its technical approval by the FDA. "You have to go to war with [FDA] for the best prelaunch labeling!" he insisted, articulating a stunning new role for PR as drug-labeling experts. And no more shilly-shallying about the drug's biggest selling point. "You have to get aggressive about creating a unique market segment that you can tightly control. I mean, like in the case of BuSpar. It wasn't good enough to launch it as a drug for anxiety. We had to go back and relaunch it for *persistent* anxiety!" This prelaunch PR would only be truly effective if you "dominate the promotional arena to win extraordinary early awareness — you must bombard them weekly to launch it properly!" He gave the example of the prostate drug Flomax: some 70 percent of the company's total promotional budget was spent during the first ninety days of its launch. Lilly, too, was spending millions on prelaunch public relations for duloxetine, or Cymbalta, its next antidepressant, even though it had not yet been approved by the FDA.

Perhaps the most striking transformation was taking place in the way big pharma viewed its relationship with patient advocacy groups, everything from the National Mental Health Foundation to the Psoriasis Foundation. In the past, pharma had used its sponsorship of such organizations as a way to raise awareness of certain conditions and perhaps to give a nudge, through patient testimony, to a flagging new drug application during FDA advisory committee meetings. The old patient organization sponsorships, when it got right down to it, were "a way to clean up your image," explained David Stern, the director of reproduc-

tive marketing for Organon International. Such were most helpful because "third-party groups are able to make statements that
pharma is not allowed to due to the regulatory climate." But now
that the Supreme Court had rendered that reason moot, there
were other, more pointed uses for patient organization sponsorship. "Increasingly, patient organizations are a way that a patient
chooses a physician and medications," Stern explained.

And they were open to pharma leadership. Stern told his own
story as a bellwether. Although he was head of Organon's marketing of infertility drugs, he had no problem securing a place on
the board of directors of the American Infertility Association
(AIA). This he did slowly. "Don't hard-sell it," he cautioned. Instead "offer them something that they can suggest corrections
on" and "have a sit-down" with their locals. "Don't insist that
you have to brand their Web site" in return for your dollars. Instead take the longer road, as he did. When Organon completed
an infertility drug study, Stern convinced the AIA to endorse it.
That made it possible for Organon to get the study posted on
a nonprofit Internet site. It elicited 12 million responses. That
built credibility for the company and its drugs because "the patient advocates are considered to be unbiased." In other words,
Organon purchased the perception of objectivity, and the patient's attention, for a study that may well have been objective
in the first place.

A little later, wending one's way to the PMC luncheon, an at-
tendee might have asked, Well, all of those ideas are great, but
how can my company try them out? The answer was right on the
conference floor in the PMC display booths. There, state-of-the-
art software companies hawked programs that used e-mail to detail physicians. Old-style radio networks showed how pharma
could use the airwaves to reach millions of specific radio audiences, everything from the "youth buy," to "urban contemporar-
ies," to the "African American buy," to the "women's buy." One
troublingly named company, Blitz Research, touted its abilities
not to target doctors directly, but rather nurses and physicians'
assistants, who, monitored by supervising physicians, write
more than 730 million prescriptions a year. ("Do you know

which nurse practitioners and physicians' assistants write prescriptions under your targeted audience? We do!") There were companies that specialized simply in creating "disease starter kits" for patients or jumbo posters for firms that did health care communications. In one ad for a company called Commonhealth, an attractive young woman in a yoga pose was shown juggling a stream of giant pill granules pouring out of a huge capsule; the "balls" were emblazoned with such scientifically technical words as "hope," "ideas," "belief," and "branding." Below her appeared perhaps the most concrete philosophical mission statement for the newly synergized era yet: "Commonhealth Confession #5," it began: "The truth: the message is part of the medicine." It then went on:

> Can healthcare communication influence healthcare outcomes? Does branding enhance the placebo effect? Our take on it? We believe image and information, imagination and belief, play a huge role in the healing process. Feeding their minds can fuel positive change in both physicians and patients. Within the healthcare marketing arena, you'll find thousands of people sincerely motivated by the desire to improve health and save lives. Communicators committed to delivering messages that are truly part of the medicine. That constitutes a psychic bottom line that few other industries pursue.

Further on was the unassuming star of the demo floor, a congenial, engaging woman named Pat Procopio, director of marketing for IMS, the health data giant. Procopio, a former schoolteacher who had been attracted to health care marketing for many of the same idealistic reasons that attracted her to teaching, demonstrated a new piece of software, sold to top pharmaceutical executives. It was called the Prescriber Profiler. The Profiler used traditional Intercontinental Marketing Service (IMS) data — the kind that Merck and Pfizer had found so helpful in the 1990s — and combined it with a new kind of information, known as patient-level data. This information was purchased from a wide variety of new players on the health care scene — everyone from HMOs to employers to labs to medical specialists. The patient name was, as required by law, blanked out. But these suppliers had replaced the blanks with encrypted numbers. That allowed a specific patient to be tracked anonymously through several health care experiences; his transactions were then merged with prescription data, then with payer data. Millions of Americans were now leaving behind, unbeknownst to them, very distinct and traceable pharma identities — the only thing missing from that identity was name, address, and phone number. In the Prescriber Profiler, IMS took this data and merged it with its huge log of information on specific physicians.

The result was a pharma CEO's joy ride. As Procopio demonstrated, a marketing executive concerned about whether a new drug was finding the right new customers could now "drill down" at will to all kinds of populations. One could simply type in the name of, say, Dr. R. K. Smith of Los Angeles, California, followed by a wide variety of other parameters: Zocor, 91104 Zip Code, male, number of refills, beta-blockers. What would pop up on the screen was every one of Dr. Smith's patients, sans name, who fit that description; that is, all the guys over forty on my block who'd been on Merck's cholesterol medication who also had high blood pressure and who were taking a competitor's med for that. Those would be perfect candidates for a switch campaign to the Prescriber Profiler executive's new blood pressure drug. Sales reps could then be primed to target Dr. Smith with as many special incentives and patient educational programs as possible. The Profiler gave the drug executive a desk-to-doctor's-brain pipeline undreamed of in the past. Drilling down — Bill Steere's dream — had merged with the Internet's ability to store huge amounts of data and then make it personal. If Jan Leschly could see it all now.

Away from confabs like the PMC, a new generation of health care communicators was completely retooling what it meant to be in pharma marketing. Nowhere was their new work better viewed than in the burgeoning pharmaceuticals trade press. Once confined to a few monthlies and newsletters, the pharma press exploded with amazing accounts of e-detailing, Internet-supported product launches, and, most sexy of all, tales of compliance and persistence. Mission accomplished! If the cutting-edge technical and creative talent had been inclined toward software and "e-tailing" a few years before, now the hipsters were in pharma, screw all that eBay action. At the ultrahip Art Center College of Design in Pasadena, California, once known for its auto and product design department, one of the hottest new fields was . . . pharmaceutical graphics. In the world of exhibit development (as in museum and educational exhibits), pharma had become a major new source of money to some of the hottest young design shops. One remarkable example was a whiz-bang science exhibit, "Brain: The World Inside Your Head," making the rounds of the nation's science museums. It was entirely funded by Pfizer. Although it was a well-rounded show, it made no bones about slipping in the company's view of what caused a number of diseases that affect the brain, including the questionable notion that "depression may be caused by an imbalance of neurotransmitters."

Big pharma's growing "teaching" function played large at major medical association conferences. At the 2002 meeting of the prestigious American Psychiatric Association, an exhibit by the makers of a powerful drug for schizophrenia showed psychiatrists "how your patients feel." Set up inside the cavernous Moscone Center in San Francisco, the company's giant pavilions invited the curious to come in and sit down. Once inside, barraged by video, audio, and even weather-simulation machines, psychiatrists could experience how a schizophrenic who had forgotten to take his meds might feel when riding a public bus. There were sudden stops and starts; air blew in their faces; visuals were distorted. What, exactly, this demonstration sought to impart in terms of medical information was unclear. But those who experienced it received, once more, reinforcement about which drug might prevent it from happening to their patients.

The teaching function of big pharma focused on patients, too. The Internet was key for companies like Braun Consulting. According to one of its executives, the Web "offers a unique platform for creating deep, profitable relationships between brand managers, patients, and physicians." What do patients get out of it? According to Braun, all kinds of things, like "a script with which to better communicate with their doctor." The script included such queries as "So, doctor, is [prescription drug X] right for me?" It did not include, "Is there a generic version of that?" The company also provided patients with "mentor-peers" and a good old disease starter kit.

Physicians, of course, had always been subject to, and often profited intellectually from, all kinds of learning and reference materials from pharmaceuticals companies. And most physicians, as they age and gain wisdom, learn how to use such perks to the patient's advantage, deducting the hype and using the science to a good end. But in recent years the industry unleashed such a flood of sponsored materials that it was difficult to tell where pharma ended and where independent medicine stood. To wit, the industry now provided 57 percent of the revenue for the nation's 686 *accredited* continuing medical education (CME) providers, a whopping $720 million in 2002 alone.

In medical schools, where pharma had always plied for early brand loyalty with free stethoscopes and black bags, the detailing turned more intellectually intimate. Now the industry routinely sponsored journal clubs, where young doctors learn how to review new data, and paid for weekly speakers on crucial medical issues. As the psychiatrist and professor Dan Shapiro wrote in the *New York Times,* obviously distressed, "Sales reps enjoy full access to our mailboxes and regularly detail our trainees in their offices, hallways, and in our little [staff] kitchen."

In the realm of event marketing, itself perhaps the biggest growth category overall, Pfizer again led the way. For the debut of its new migraine pill, Relpax, the company converted a wing of New York's Grand Central Station into a spa, or, as its designers put it, "a soothing oasis of the senses." There was a three-piece chamber orchestra, yoga clinics, free massages, gourmet food, and a Zen garden, where no one, apparently, was supposed to contemplate who was ultimately paying for it all. Relpax is indicated only for the treatment of the symptoms of migraine and, as only a small percentage of headaches are migraines, one might have wondered who else — upscale regular headache sufferers? — would benefit from the spa message.

Then there was Glaxo and its new asthma drug, Advair. Glaxo had worked hard to brand the drug in a populist way, hiring racecar great Bobby Labonte to be its spokesman and setting up Advair demo booths at big stock car rallies all over the United States. But Advair sales lagged. The company turned to the Grey Healthcare Group, a division of one of the most powerful ad agencies in the world. Grey's director of services, Tom O'Dell, had a keen grasp of his customers. As he explained to one trade magazine, his team came to see that "the emotional space or territory a brand owns is every bit as important as the clinical story it needs to tell. The insight into that emotional need is the hook that, at the end of the day, makes the doctor feel 'this is the brand that really understands all of my needs.'" But how to find out what the doctor thinks he needs? At first Glaxo thought the hook was convenience — Advair was easy for patients to take because it delivered two medications at once. But as O'Dell found out, "There was another drug out there that already owned convenience." In other words, doctors didn't need another asthma drug that was convenient, a major bummer for a drug manufacturer that had pinned its hopes on that.

So what else did doctors want? To find out, O'Dell and his staff convinced a number of physicians to create "collages depicting their feelings" toward asthma. "In doing so," O'Dell recalled, "we discovered a deep sense of exasperation over compliance issues . . . We asked them, 'What does success look like?' And in words and graphics the doctors told us, in effect, 'Give me a drug that is going to make treatment success a reality.' The underlying emotional need is that doctors want to feel inspired and heroic in their treatment of patients." Although one might have surmised that without spending tens of millions of dollars that would eventually be charged back to the consumer in the form of high prices, consider what Grey came up with: a campaign image centered on one man, clad in hip waders, catching a fish. "This is George," the ad ran. "Now that his airway inflammation and bronchospasm are being effectively treated, the prize is within reach." Sales of Glaxo's drug ran to $2 billion that year. A coun-termessage might have been: This is why your Advair is so expensive that you'll have to start foraging for all your own protein in order to afford it.

These new "coping images," million-dollar versions of the dream Arthur Hull Hayes was almost pilloried for — and which the industry itself only twenty years before saw as a threat to the doctor-patient relationship — now came to dominate product launches. Consider the campaign for Effexor XR, the new version of Wyeth's successful antidepressant. The company goal was twofold: find a way to justify its higher price and create new markets along the way. One solution was to make the drug appear "young." To rev up the sales force, the company hired a rap group to pound out an "inspirational" rap battle, à la the film 8 Mile, to set the tone. It then produced a commercial that portrayed a patient asking himself, "Are you really where you want to be?" and realizing, as its creator commented, that "a greater state of improvement was possible." AstraZeneca went through a similar process with its expensive new anti-heartburn medication, Nexium. The old GERD threat wasn't enough to justify the cost anymore, as its own thought leaders told the company upon initial launch. So AstraZeneca turned up the threat — and anxiety — potential. Now the health issue wasn't GERD but actual esophageal erosion, something that happens in very few cases of true GERD, of which there are few in the first place. As one trade magazine put it, "AstraZeneca actually had to teach the market all over again to look for different issues." Actually!

There was another arena where such enterprising thought processes might be of enormous assistance to big pharma, and it had nothing at all to do with compliance and persistence. Or even with approved drugs that were deemed safe and effective. That area was clinical trials for experimental drugs and the recruitment of subjects to participate in them. Ever since the late 1980s, the costs of these FDA-required tests had soared. The industry initially attempted to deal with the problem by turning to private contract researchers outside the university system that had

traditionally been the arbiter of most trials. The thinking was
that outside the slow and methodical realm of academic organizations, pharma would have a better chance of getting more trial
designs approved and carried out. That was true. By 2000, the
great majority of clinical trials were conducted outside the academy by contract research organizations, or CROs. Some of these
firms were driven by solid scientific taskmasters with strong
managerial instincts. Some were not. Whatever their credentials, privatized clinical trials had become a boom industry in itself.

In fact, there were so many trials going on that, by the late
1990s, finding enough qualified patients — a.k.a. research subjects — was becoming increasingly expensive and time-consum-
ing. For CEOs, it became a competitive issue not unlike that of
generic drugs. A company's ability to recruit patients became a
highly visible indicator — to investors, Wall Street, and board
members — of a pharma firm's viability. If a lack of such ability
ate into the company's production of a steady stream of blockbuster drugs, it could depress stock prices and create intense
pressure by stockholders and board members. The issue was becoming an obstacle in the path of innovation and profits, at least
as seen by top executives in all major pharmaceutical companies. As the industry bible, *Pharmaceutical Executive*, put it:
"Nearly 80 percent of all clinical studies for new products fail to
finish on time, and 20 percent of those are delayed six months or
longer. It translates into a loss of $1 million a day in unrealized
sales . . . Clinical trials are the weak link in the drug pipeline
and *must be accelerated* to improve corporate growth and profitability."

They must be accelerated. In the executive suites, many believed one way to increase the chances of a new drug's success
was branding a product before it was launched. This process, also
known as "pre-prelaunch branding," involved the hiring of eminent researchers in the medical specialty into which the experimental drug fell. Those thought leaders would be consulted all
along the path to an NDA, and they would be free to talk and
write about what they heard to their peers and in journal articles.

It was a way of encouraging consensus by people who mattered, *before approval.* With the new off-label ruling, it was easy to do. In early 2003 one of the biggest New York public relations firms began promoting — only with studies, of course — Lilly's new antidepressant Cymbalta, which was still in trials, whispering whenever they passed it to influential journalists in the financial press that it was "only a matter of months" before it would be approved, which it was not.

The practice was not limited to sexy psychiatric drugs. Brad Thompson, the executive in charge of a pneumonia drug launch at Wyeth, laid the essentials bare: "A multifunctional team should be established in three to four years prelaunch to transcend mere medical and marketing coordination." In other words, to create a brand while the drug was still under study. Tim Walbert, the vice president and general manager for immunology at Abbott Labs, put it another way: "Marketing and commercial development work together and are involved in protocol development [the scientific method of the clinical trial] for phase one [human safety] and phase two [small-scale human efficacy] trials, not just for phase three [large-scale efficacy studies]." Why was that? Because "many key thought-leader perceptions of your brand will be defined during those early days." Of course, an unreconstructed purist might view these tactics as tainting the greater pool of scientific opinion, but such was not the concern, or the perceived area of responsibility, for modern pharma.

Many top executives, thinking outside the box, believed the industry's growing relations with patient advocacy groups also could help recruit more trial subjects. If such organizations were good for persistence and compliance marketing, they might be good for clinical trial recruitment. As Jeff Winter, the vice president of global public relations for Pharmacia, explained to one trade magazine, "Gone are the days when companies just handed out big checks to groups with no discussion afterward. Now we seek opportunities with groups that not only help them achieve their goals and objectives, but also help us move our businesses along."

Yet patient groups were not fast enough either. The patient-recruiting concern began trickling into the marketing and media community. The question became: How could marketing be used for patient recruitment? Slowly, a new breed of clinical trial player emerged, men and women who traveled under the title of "health care communications consultants." They specialized not in the implementation of precise scientific protocols — the main task of any clinical trial operator — but in patient recruitment, communication, and finding ways to make sure that fewer patients dropped out of costly trials. They were performance enhancers — expensive outside goads and coaches brought in by pharma to make sure that clinical trials stayed on track. They were fast, costly, and agile. Rubbing shoulders with the heads of research of the top pharma firms in the world, these communications gurus began to exert a pull on pharma's traditionally independent scientific chiefs. They were literally having lunch with them.

A most remarkable example of this synergy in big science was on display not long ago, at a research and development drug summit, held by the influential trade magazine publisher Karl Engel, at a plush Arizona resort in February 2004. Gathered around the topic of "How to Build and Maintain a Winning [New Drug] Pipeline," the meeting attracted the research and development heads of the most powerful pharmaceutical companies in the world, including Pfizer, AstraZeneca, Merck, and Lilly. There were the predictable slide show presentations, basically show-and-tells of coming drug breakthroughs. The head of R&D for Merck explained how genetics was influencing drug development, but refused to answer questions about why Vioxx was turning out to be less safe and less effective than initially promoted. (The drug was withdrawn eight months later.) The deputy chief of Lilly's R&D announced that Cymbalta would be approved any day but did not talk about emerging safety problems with the drug.

But the showstopper was a presentation not by a lone science executive and his nerdy data charts, but by a pair of gentlemen, Malcolm Bohm, the director of clinical trials for Novartis, and Frank Kilpatrick, the head of a firm called Healthcare Communications Group, who, under the topic "Clinical Trials Improve-ment," presented what they called "A Radical Proposal." The star was clearly Kilpatrick.

Frank Kilpatrick had been kicking around the advertising and marketing scene since the early 1980s, when he was billed as a whiz kid for struggling media firms. He had worked at all the hot agencies, from Grey Advertising to Knapp to Whittle. He was an intense fellow, Californian in mien with Robert Redford hair and a young Gary Busey countenance. He had no formal medical training, nor, for the most part, did the rest of his staff, coming, as they did, respectively, from a TV production outfit, a helicop-ter company, and a firm that sold endoscopes. But he seemed to understand how to improve clinical trial recruitment *outcomes*, and that is what attracted pharma.

The key to Kilpatrick's radical proposal, he proclaimed as Novartis's Bohm looked on, was to use all of the tools of the modern communications industry to predict which patient re-cruitment methods would work best. "We have to understand — really get wet in the field with patients and drill down," he said. Why? Because "50 percent of prescreenings fail because of 'no in-terest' [a little box checked on surveys] by subjects. So the task is, 'How do we gain interest by patients?'" (Of course, the task might also be, now that they had said no, Why don't we leave them alone, but that was not in the radical proposal.) The answer was the strategic use of communications consultants who un-derstood what messages motivated people and how to measure success. After all, Kilpatrick said, when you cut through all the gobbledygook about protocols and patient subpopulations, suc-cess in clinical trial recruitment meant one thing: How many pa-tients make it all the way through a trial?

To that end, Kilpatrick demonstrated how the new technolo-gies of data mining and on-line tracking could identify which clinical investigator sites had hit their recruiting targets most of-ten, then steer patients to those sites. Communications consul-tants — Kilpatrick, for example — could act as "mentors" to site managers who were "in nonalignment," New Age–speak for not hitting their target numbers. They could conduct what Kilpatrick called "rescue mode" campaigns for flagging recruitment sites, even constructing patient focus groups to determine which messages were working and which were not. That kind of internal self-feedback loop — interacting with subjects while a trial was in process — might raise eyebrows in traditional scientific and university circles. It was thus no surprise that Kilpatrick believed that private-sector CROs were almost always the way to go. "Academic entities," he said, "might not provide a real-world assist." No, probably not. Database mining worked with patient recruitment in another way. By accessing information from patient advocacy groups and previous clinical trials, consultants could identify patients who had been "compliant" — they had successfully completed the experiment, done all the follow-up interviews, blood work, and lab tests necessary to qualify for the study's exacting protocol. To CROs, they were pure gold.

Using such techniques, Kilpatrick said, allowed one to understand what motivated patients. But where, literally, to find the patients? In this Kilpatrick was surprisingly blunt: among the poor and underserved. The poor, of course, have always been disproportionately represented in clinical trials, just as they are disproportionately underserved in health care generally; clinical trials are one way for them to make a small amount of money, usually in the form of a stipend. And trials are, when all is said and done, a way for them to get medical attention and services that they cannot afford. You really did not have to recruit them. They came.

But Kilpatrick said those days were over. Now, he said, pharma needed to invest more money in finding and recruiting even the poor into their trials. They were not, obviously, going to be found via the Internet. Pharma had to do things like "deploying clinical fieldworkers to locate marginalized patients where they live and receive treatment: hospitals, board and care facilities, drop-in centers, soup kitchens." There were other places to find them as well: at YMCAs, in low-income churches, and by networking through the home health care programs of community hospitals.

Kilpatrick was then able to show how such tactics had worked in "saving" one large company's launch of a new drug for major depression disorder. "At an approximate cost of $600,000, the rescue recruitment program gained 125 new randomized clinical-trial patients . . . and brought the study in on schedule. Without the agency's assistance, the study would have been delayed by 8.6 months. Estimating the product's first-year sales at $20 million a month, the investment had the potential to yield the sponsor $159 million in revenue." And that, Kilpatrick did not say, was really getting wet.

The excesses of marketing-speak, of course, are always fun to poke at, but no one should underestimate what, exactly, such speak means. It means that more money is spent on the *acceleration* of new drugs, many of which are not large improvements over existing drugs, and on promoting that drug before it is approved. What the cumulative effect of spending billions on that process means for the medical and health culture as a whole is not apparent, but one thing is clear: increasingly, Dr. Joe and Dr. Jane Average are being pulled into the process. The lure, says Alison MacPherson, president of a CRO named Pharmbrite, in Los Angeles, is basic. "One, the money. HMOs have so restricted the ability to make money that [clinical trials are] one way [for physicians] to increase the flow," she says. Doctors get paid for running the trials and simply for referring patients into them. "Two, the status. It is a way they can feel powerful, or authoritative, again. It puts them back in touch with their science side, and with the status of that."

The branding, the PR, the money — whatever the reason — by 2004, when the research group CenterWatch published a survey called "Will Physicians Refer Their Patients into Clinical Trials?" physicians were in deep alignment with pharma's drive for more research subjects. "One third of clinical trial volunteers report that they learned about a clinical trial through their primary or specialty physician," the journal reported. Even more, 39 percent, came because of something they saw or heard in the media ads, and 28 percent came because of ads by CROs.

All across the United States, patient recruitment throve. At the high end, one might see ads at places like the cafeteria at UCLA Medical Center, part of one of the world's most prestigious medical schools. Up on a corkboard there, one read: "Free Social Skills Training for Kids. Does your child need help making and keeping friends? If so, your child may be able to join a UCLA research study. Free pizza and parking" and "Child Anxiety Study. Is your child afraid to go to school . . . overly worried about bad things . . . afraid to be away from you? If so, your child may be suffering from an anxiety disorder." There were studies, using drugs or placebos, for kids who experienced separation anxiety at summer camp and for depression. At the low end, appeals were more direct. In the large-circulation *LA Weekly*, snuggled along-side ads touting "Learn the art of massage" and "Are you a single gorgeous woman with an amazing body between the ages of 25– 34 who wants to be pampered by a wealthy gentleman?" ran the following: "Depressed? No insurance? You may be able to par-ticipate in our study of an investigational antidepressant medi-cation combination, with up to $600 compensation, free study medication, free physical and mental health exam, and study-related laboratory testing."

The point is not that clinical trials are not important, nor that the physicians involved in them are not, in the main, skillful, caring men and women who are primarily interested in getting their patients well. They are, and they are. The point is that these trials are also commercial endeavors, now more than ever, with nonmedical aims thrumming below the surface. They are part of a sales machine, which has, in the language of clinical trials, a very different endpoint indeed.

For just a moment — but for just a moment — let us pause here and take a breath. OK, now let us cut everyone just a little — only a little — slack. In the modern world of service and culture industries, an increasingly large chunk of Americans work in jobs that benefit from creative marketing. There is a man or a woman, one hopes several, who will be assigned to find many creative ways to sell this book. That person will take the concept and then find audiences to which it might appeal, then tilt the campaign in those directions. The same might be done with the latest brand of chocolate chip cookie, deodorant, low-carb beer, or cell phone. The genius and the insanity of our system run like that, and most of us participate in it, for better and for worse.

Yet in the case of pharmaceuticals, we are talking about something fundamentally different. These are potent, sophisticated chemical compounds, developed at the cost of hundreds of millions of dollars, vetted by leading scientists for safety, and then very carefully indicated for use *only* with the supervision of a physician. *These products actually change our body.* Yes, actually. And they are not like consumer goods for another reason: We have to have them. We have only one body. Our demand for keeping it healthy is inelastic. We have to take these products because *they are prescribed by an expert* so that we can live better, longer. In the case of pharma, one consistent question arrives with the frequency of an errant cousin at just the wrong social moment: Is the pill worth it? To find out, one might first ask, What is the full extent of pharmaceutical tribesmanship in America today, and what are the impulses, social and otherwise, that tribal marketing exploits?

WHY OPEN OUR MOUTH?

And so, Why do we take the pills? In the most primal sense, it is because they are there, and because we are human. Pharmaceuticals, just like most forms of technology, represent humankind's unique inclination to shape both personal and collective destiny. Pills are an escape from fate, via science, logic, and will. Yet the way we view pills has changed, some would say radically, in the past few decades. Whereas in the past, the (legal) pharmaceutical escape from fate was mainly about curing disease and infection, it now encompasses and justifies itself on the more general notion of health, and on the more particular concept of chronic disease. Health now means different things to different people: it can mean a state of well-being, an absence of disease, a lowered risk profile. It is, to many, an unattainable ideal. Health, it has been observed by more than one modern philosopher, is the new God.

One can witness this phenomenon in a million ways, but perhaps the best is by looking at how health — and what might be called health literacy — has affected God, once the ultimate arbiter of fate. Consider two of the Seven Deadly Sins. In the battle against obesity and the chronic diseases that flow from it, talking about gluttony and sloth — the overconsumption of calories from food and the underexpenditure of calories from sitting on one's rump — will, today, get you exactly one thing: an egg in the face for stigmatizing people. Science shows that getting fat is not simply due to eating too many doughnuts or OD'ing on TV. It is about genes and about environment, about social class and status. But ask just about any public health expert or obesity scholar what should be done about slowing the trend, and you will get the same answer. We have to get people to stop making "imprudent lifestyle choices." In other words, we have to help people to stop being gluttonous and slothful, without saying so. This isn't to suggest that we should go back to using the Seven Deadlies as a guiding paradigm. It is simply recognition of one deep current of modern medical culture.

What about God and psychiatric medicine? Though theirs has never been a happy marriage, particularly in the more conservative realms of American Christianity, you would never know it nowadays on Christian drive-time radio. On any day in Dallas, for example, one can tune in to a popular radio show called *New Life Live* and hear dialogues between Dr. Paul Meier, the show's host, and a variety of traditional Christians in psychological pain. One day a few years ago, a young woman called in to ask for advice regarding her abusive, philandering boyfriend. The exchange went something like this:

CALLER: . . . and there's really nothing I can do about him and his porn [*crying*]. The man is a porn addict, like all men these days, with their Internet and all —

MEIER: Slow down, Donna, slow down. You can't do anything about the Internet, can you — ?

CALLER: Well, no, but —

MEIER: And this isn't just about him, now is it?

CALLER: I've had abusive relationships before —

MEIER: So what I'm going to ask you, Donna, is are you willing to give me a try, a good try, so that you can get out of this cycle of anger, depression, and self-destruction?

CALLER: Eh, yes, I guess?

MEIER: You guess? Yes or no!

CALLER: Yes. Definitely! It's what Jesus would want —

MEIER: That's right, Donna. That *is* what Jesus would want. He'd want you to read — and I want you to treat this as a prescription, I'm a doctor, remember — I want you to every night, in your prayers, I want you to read Philippians 4:6. In it, and I will read it for you right now, we learn this: "Be anxious for nothing, but in everything by prayer . . . let your requests be known to God, and the peace of God, which surpasses all comprehension, shall guard your hearts and minds in Jesus Christ."

CALLER: OK, doctor —

MEIER: Wait! Wait! That's not all! Donna, do you have a family physician? I'm sure you do. So go get a pen and paper and write this down. Tell him you want Effexor — that's an antidepressant, one time a day for a week, then twice a day. Then ask him for some Wellbutrin — that's an antianxiety aid — and I want you to take one hundred fifty milligrams a day, with the Effexor. Then be sure to schedule a visit with him in another month.

CALLER: What if that doesn't work?

MEIER: Then call me back, Donna. I'm here every day . . .

If the exchange sounds strange to non-Evangelicals, it should, for to say that modern psychiatry and modern Evangelical Christianity do not mix is like saying that the weather in Burma is often very warm. As recently as the early 1990s, the Reverend Jerry Falwell joined with Scientology to protest the onslaught of Prozac. In doing so Falwell had sounded the traditional Evangelic objection to modern psychopharmacology: it was, he said, a stalking-horse for secular paganism, offering a biological excuse for moral failings and insufficient Christian joyfulness.

Yet today, Meier's program, which now has one hundred radio affiliates, is hardly off the grid. In fact, it and its imitators — and they are many — represent the basics of the growing Christian Counseling Movement, which was begun by a series of enlightened Christian physicians out of Duke University in the late 1970s. The basics of the movement, as spelled out in *New Life*

Live's "Statement of Faith," include a belief in "humanity's depravity," that "the Bible is the only infallible, inerrant word of God," and that "all psychiatric principles should be thoroughly evaluated through the Scriptures." And that includes a whole shelf of the once verboten pharmaceuticals. The movement has garnered millions of followers in major cities around the country. Meier's Christian Therapist Network alone fields some 20,000 calls a month, often referring callers to his own New Life Clinics, where they can get spiritual and pharmacological help for everything from depression to sexual addiction to panic disorder and obsessive-compulsive disorder.

Already some of the founders of the movement are wondering if Meier and his imitators have gone too far. By embracing modern pharmacology, Christian Counseling may have also lost something special, they worry. As Dan Blazer, a professor of psychiatry at Duke University and a Christian Counseling founder himself, says, "Psychiatry and Christianity have never experienced better superficial relations. Each has accommodated the other. So the tension between them, which should stimulate advances in our understanding of our deepest emotional pains, has given way to a comfortable segmentation of the brain from the soul."

What might loosely be called the "health media" also figures into the social equation surrounding Generation Rx. There are those, following in the footsteps of Ivan Illich, who would even make the case that today's constant bombardment of often conflicting health messages makes us more likely to become ill. Such observers point to the rapid rise of the health media itself. Until twenty years ago, no American newspaper had beat reporters assigned to the strange notion of personal health. Now they are legion, and their sections are profitable, laden with ads for everything from clinical trials to breast augmentation.

But does heightened awareness of health dangers really make people sick? One would think that such a topic might occupy a central concern of modern health studies, but in the United States such is not the case. Dr. Keith Petrie, a professor in the health psychology department at the University of Auckland,

New Zealand, has long been fascinated by how patients view modernity — that is, how suspicious they are of modern life. His work centers on "health worry," everything from concerns about cell phones to environmental toxins to genetically modified foods. He has found a consistent connection between the degree to which a person worries about such things and individual complaints to doctors about chronic fatigue syndrome and food intolerance. As he notes, this phenomenon is relatively new. "The media's increased coverage of health topics, in stories on the dangers lurking in ordinary activities such as air travel and vaccination, has raised worries about routine health care and increased people's perception of their vulnerability to new and exotic diseases. Media stories also tend to misrepresent the dangers of new environmental influences and aspects of modernity, while playing down more mundane causes of ill health, such as the link between tobacco and heart disease. *This focus of the media on risks with a novelty value fosters the belief that they are far more common than they actually are* [my italics]." The result, he concludes, is that "people now feel much more vulnerable."

Yet the real reasons people seek help and use prescription drugs for chronic disease are at once more concrete, complex, and daunting than at first or second glance. Still, if we consider how pharma has chosen to market most new products, the view becomes a little clearer. Almost all chronic-disease drugs are sold because they increase performance, sustain productivity, lessen pain, or increase longevity. They are all, in a sense, drugs for a work-based culture.

And work in twenty-first-century America, as anyone save the most insulated among us know too well, is no predictable beast. In contrast to the experience of the immediate postwar generation, work life today is, to paraphrase Hobbes, nasty, brutish, and short — after, of course, some vaunted period of amazing creativity and optimism. (It is also air-conditioned and heated, a good thing.) One reason for the stress is clear: rapid and constant organizational change. It is a force so intrinsic to modern work life that it has remade the very notion of work. The three principal virtues of the earlier generation — dedication, specialization, and loyalty — have been replaced by three new attributes — networking, flexibility, and constant reeducation. And new expectations: the average work year for prime-age working couples has increased by at least one hundred hours in the last two decades. Just like pharma CEOs, we are increasingly conscious of our performance in almost all areas of our lives, and with that increased consciousness comes a toll on body, mind, and spirit. High levels of emotional exhaustion are the norm for 25 to 30 percent of the workforce.

To simplify, it may be that our love-hate relationship with prescription drugs for chronic illness has a rational adaptive function: in ways we cannot yet express, they help us through a new work world. It is a world that has changed under our feet, one in which we are expected to accommodate change — quickly — or be left behind.

But what do we know, in terms of hard data, about modern work? Unfortunately, the status of occupational health in America is beggarly at best, strange for a nation at the edge of redefining work itself. Today, mention occupational health and you will be accused of being a regulation freak, an overprotective nanny, someone selling safety equipment, or the author of a plot by unnamed liberals who want to reestablish the hegemony of organized labor and "destroy" our competitive edge. Whereas we need a new Ramazzini, the Renaissance Italian who invented occupational medicine, we get, instead, labor secretaries who are uninterested in labor itself. The one ongoing U.S. survey of changes in work organization and their health impact was discontinued in the early 1980s, despite its oft cited usefulness by business and government.

The Swedes, as well as a number of other economically advanced nations (and many not so), get the workplace-health issue, at least on a conceptual level. Following a severe recession in the early 1990s, they began to study long-term absence from jobs due to sickness, hospital admissions, and workplace instability. The initial findings were somewhat predictable. People who worked in companies that were downsizing tended to be sicker, absent longer, and in hospital more often than those in firms and organizations that kept the status quo. The increase was largely blamed on personnel cuts and overly lean organizations.

Later findings, however, blew the researchers' minds. Looking at changes during an economic *expansion*, when productivity boomed and joblessness decreased, they found similar rates of increased sickness. "All forms of organizational instability, including rapid expansion, were associated with both higher job strain and higher levels of risk for cardiovascular disease," they wrote. In their final study, published in *The Lancet* in 2004, they got to the heart of the problem: "Repeated exposure to rapid personnel expansion, possibly connected with centralization of functions, statistically predicts long-term sickness, absence, and hospital admissions." What was at the root? Something familiar to most American workers: "higher turnover, more individual (as opposed to collective) demands, and differences in organizational climate and managerial style." White-collar workers seemed to fare the worst, particularly in rapidly growing companies. In a separate study, the authors linked job expansion to increases in specific risk and disease categories. Employees in growing small firms — the kind celebrated in every business.com magazine around the world — registered unexpected shifts in their health profiles, with higher cholesterol, triglyceride, and fibrinogen levels, all of which are associated with an increased risk of heart disease.

How might we digest such research? In one way it is merely confirmatory. Most of us have lived the modern work life and made our pact with it. But what if that pact is driving chronic disease? What if the modern philosophy of work, and particularly that of the modern reengineered company — demanding of endless "flexibility" and ever increasing productivity while simultaneously promoting the idea that employees should tolerate ambiguity and not expect any security — is a new and little understood source of modern illness? Work, work, work, and bend your life around it. It's a philosophy that inflects the nation's three major pharmaceutical tribes.

GEN-RX1: THE TRIBE OF HIGH-PERFORMANCE YOUTH

The oldest of today's pharmaceutical tribes is, paradoxically, made up of the young. It is the tribe of Ritalin and attention deficit hyperactivity disorder (ADHD, usually just referred to as ADD). The tribe includes as its membership an estimated 5 million children and adolescents, along with untold millions of supportive family members. It is, in essence, Gen-Rx1. It is arguably one of the most well-developed pharma tribes, possessing, as it does, deeply held beliefs about the cause and treatment of the disease as well as a vast trove of taboos, all underwritten, either directly or indirectly, by the new nexus of pharma, patient organizations, and incentivized physicians. That it is a pharma-driven tribe does not mean that ADD is not a real disorder, or that Ritalin does not help those who suffer from it. Respectively, it is, and it does, at least in the short term. But it does mean that the tribe is also part of two other phenomena: the overprescription of drugs, in this case Ritalin and its competitors, as well as the overly narrow "consensus" about ADD's cause and treatment. And these, whether by intent or design, almost always accrue to the benefit of pharma's bottom line.

The short history: Ritalin, or methylphenidate, was first synthesized by European researchers in the 1940s. It was part of an effort to find a nonaddictive stimulant. The effort, like similar ones directed at finding nonaddictive painkillers, failed. Ritalin as we know it today is, as then, a stimulant with many of the same chemical structures, metabolic processes, potentially addictive qualities, and clinical effects as amphetamines. Although initially approved in the United States in 1957 to treat medication-induced lethargy, it was soon marketed by its maker, Ciba-Geigy, as a treatment for impaired memory among geriatric patients. This was because Ritalin, like most stimulants, had long been known for its ability to do more than simply speed up the lethargic. It also improved performance. This trick it achieved via a complex chain of chemical events that begins with raising blood pressure. Like other stimulants, Ritalin's most pronounced effect was that it seemed to intensify a patient's focus.

People who took it were able to concentrate better. Its outward manifestations were odd: adults who took it seemed to get agitated and hyper; kids who took it seemed to become calm. As it would turn out, both responses came from the same focus-intensifying effect. Children, particularly overactive ones who had behavior problems, simply experienced intensified focus as calmative; their parents experienced their children's change as one of containing often self-destructive bursts of manic energy. Although there had long been anecdotal evidence that Ritalin helped various behavior problems in kids, it was not until the early 1960s that the drug, after clinical trials showed that it and another stimulant, Dexedrine, produced predictable calming effects in children, was approved by the FDA for treatment of overactive kids. Of the two drugs, Ritalin became the standard treatment for hyperactivity because, according to Lawrence Diller, the author of perhaps the most authoritative and balanced book on the subject, "It was not amphetamine." Its name did not ferry the pejorative of its more media-exposed chemical brother. Sales of Ritalin soared through the mid-1960s.

Yet Ritalin was never immune from the vicissitudes of public and medical opinion about stimulants. In the mid-sixties, its sales were affected by a scare in Sweden about Ritalin overuse. Then they recovered. In the 1970s, the first of several anti-Ritalin books appeared. At the same time the Church of Scientology launched a campaign against the drug. Sales dropped again, then recovered.

All the while, researchers were discovering new facets of the drug. Much of it centered not on Ritalin's ability to contain hyperactivity, but on its ability to improve performance. At the same time the scientific and medical academies were increasingly intrigued with something they called "attention deficits" in problem kids. Some of these children were not hyperactive at all, but had trouble concentrating and in controlling their impulses. The problem for Ciba-Geigy was that Ritalin could not be sold for such a purpose; there was no official childhood disease or disorder with attention problems as its main component, and so the company could not apply to the FDA for approval to market

Ritalin as a treatment for it. And they could not market it off label in the unenlightened patronizing era, as Judge Scalia and others might have it, of government regulation. Ritalin was thus a potential cure in search of a diagnosis.

That changed in 1980, when the American Psychiatric Association for the first time listed ADD in the *Diagnostic and Statistical Manual of Mental Disorders*, or *DSM*. The *DSM* did not list a cause for ADD. There has, in fact, never been a consensus about what causes the disorder. There was no test for it. But one thing was known: children with ADD who took Ritalin got better — sometimes dramatically and almost always for short periods of time, sometimes longer. The drug thus became the diagnosis. If one responded to Ritalin, one "had" ADD. Sales soared again, and this time one of the biggest categories of new patients consisted of children who were not hyperactive, but who had performance problems at school and behavior problems at home. Ritalin had come of age.

It had done so during the great postwar transformation of American society, one that saw women enter the workforce in unprecedented numbers, when day care became a norm, when demands for kids to perform at school and home increased, and when, simultaneously, resources — money in the case of schools, time and energy in the case of parents — grew scarcer. All of a sudden there were unprecedented numbers of kids taking Ritalin. Were more kids indeed too active, distractible, and impulsive? Or was a more anxious, work-based society, stretched for compensatory resources, no longer able to accommodate them? No one knew, and few undertook a study of such.

Then, in the mid-1980s, an unkind wind blew again for Ciba and Ritalin. The Church of Scientology began suing physicians who prescribed the drug for ADD. The media widened the debate, with its propensity for controversy accentuating long-held scholarly divisiveness about Ritalin. The result: between 1989 and 1991, sales fell by 37 percent. For the executives at Ciba, whose board had grown used to double-digit growth, the pressure was intense. Fortunately for them, they were operating in the new, post–Hatch-Waxman regime, when it was more and more acceptable, and permissible, to innovate, and when Gerry Mossinghoff at the Pharmaceutical Manufacturers Association was pointing the way, boldly.

Perhaps Ciba's most important innovation was the company's growing relationship, both through donations and other resources, with an organization known as CHADD, or Children with Attention Deficit Disorder. CHADD was, at the time of Ciba's sales crisis with Ritalin, a small but quickly growing patient advocacy group. It had been founded in 1987 by a group of parents of ADD sufferers. The group was not only concerned with helping children and parents cope with the disorder, but also with getting better educational and medical resources for those with ADD, then unrecognized as an official disability under U.S. law and hence not qualifying for special educational benefits and occupational considerations. CHADD's members quite rightly wanted their children to get their share of the pie.

In CHADD, Ciba found synergy and savior. Beginning in the early 1990s, the company began pumping hundreds of thousands of dollars into CHADD in unrestricted educational grants. That meant the little organization could spend it on whatever it wanted to spend it on, and that meant three things: spreading the word about ADD and its treatment; campaigning to get the disorder classified as a disability; and creating an ongoing interaction among parents, kids, and the ADD medical community. CHADD was phenomenally effective. Its membership roles bloomed with tens of thousands of new members, which the organization mobilized to win inclusion of ADD in the 1991 Individuals with Disabilities Education Act, or IDEA. And with that inclusion, Ciba got for Ritalin a legitimacy windfall. ADD was recognized by the government as a legal disability, making it easier for patients to get reimbursed for treatment. As Ritalin was, essentially, the diagnosis and treatment all wrapped up in one, so would IDEA become, quite simply, "the single biggest factor in the explosion of ADD diagnosis and Ritalin use in this country," writes Lawrence Diller. By the late 1990s, the United States consumed 90 percent of the world's Ritalin. The disorder was continually talked up as affecting "up to 10 percent of America's children," although many in the academy believed it was more like 3 to 5 percent.

Yet perhaps CHADD's more lasting benefit to Ciba-Geigy (now renamed Novartis) had nothing to do with law and everything to do with tribal market building — with the popularization, support, and reinforcement of beliefs and taboos about ADD and Ritalin. At the CHADD tribe's core is the assumption, still unproven, that ADD is solely a beast of biological origin. The group popularized one study in particular that showed differences in glucose metabolism in the brains of ADD kids; it did not popularize the same researcher's later findings, which were not so conclusive. Over and over, CHADD drove home the biology-only bias. Anyone who disagreed was blaming the victim. This belief flowed directly from, and reinforced, CHADD's biggest recruiting tool: its constantly repeated doctrine that the ADD parent is not at fault. The basis of that doctrine was humane and understandable, and often true. Many ADD kids came from households that were high functioning and highly empathetic, with parents that gave their all trying to provide their children with a balanced, nurturing environment; their children were, indeed, likely hard-wired for behavioral problems, and Ritalin could help in the short term.

But many ADD kids were products of the kind of homes clearly on the rise in reengineered America. Yes, the family was together, and yes, the parents were concerned and loving. But the home dynamics were tense, stretched by the demands of the new economy, the fragmenting treats of TV and video, and the underfunding of schools. To these parents, the claim that the disorder was purely biological came as enormous relief. It was a balm to the nagging notion that the fast-track life, the one you seemed to have to live to afford the best for your family, was not good for your kids. And so did the CHADD tribe become the Novartis tribe, though no one stated it quite that way.

But what was wrong with that? In some ways, nothing. Ritalin was safe, and, as research would show, it improved the performance of kids who did not have ADD as well. Yet, ironically, therein *did* reside the problem. The drug was still effectively the diagnosis. If it worked, a child had ADD. The result was rampant overprescribing of Ritalin. The drug and its imitators have become the default for almost all kids with behavior problems, just as SSRIs have become the default for adults (and increasingly kids and adolescents) with depression. And that conjures an important question: If the first instinct for all such problems is to medicate, what becomes of the environment as a possible cause? Answer: It gets ignored. There are almost no studies of ADD rates in crowded classrooms versus noncrowded classrooms, of ADD rates in families under financial distress versus those not under stress, or of ADD rates in families with a stay-at-home parent versus no stay-at-home parent — despite the fact that the best clinicians who deal with ADD almost always consider the home and school situation as critical components of prescribing a course of therapy, be it pharmacological or otherwise. Ritalin thus helps support the American work culture, where home is too often a place to get more done, more measurable things achieved, and where school is a place to prepare for that life. In one sense that is good: in the past kids with ADD ended up on the sidelines. It was simply "accepted" early on that they were not college material and were shunted aside or directed to the manual arts. Now, not only have the manual arts been defunded, but underperformance is not tolerated. We cannot afford diversity of personality, at least when it affects performance in a fairly narrow range of work-related activity.

And so in the work culture of millennial America, performance rules. It is what we invest in, and, in the case of children, Ritalin is one big channel of that investment. So, increasingly, are antidepressants, few of which have demonstrated any efficacy in clinical trials for kids but which, because of off-label marketing, are one of pharma's biggest growth categories. Spending on all forms of drugs to treat childhood and adolescent behavioral disorders rose by a whopping 77 percent between 2000 and 2003, with 65 percent of all children on such drugs taking at least one antidepressant. For the first time, drugs for childhood and adolescent mental health problems pulled ahead of antibiotics and asthma meds, the traditional market dominators in that age group. The synergy marketers boogied at full tilt. A typical advertisement in the industry trade magazine *DTC Perspectives* portrayed an attractive teen taking a study break and leaning back in her library chair. "She's not refilling her prescriptions," the ad, by a firm called RTC Relationship Marketing, said. "She says it's because she's too busy. Wouldn't you like to know the real reason?" The company could explain why.

And just what *is* happening to the first Gen-Rx, now that so many have left the nest? The earliest indications that something was different about them began to appear in the mid-1990s. To be sure, every generation of teens is labeled *different*. But previous generations were not raised in a highly pharmaceuticalized culture, a mass culture that pharma not only sells to, but also has a strong hand in creating. As such, Gen-Rx1 has all the same problems that average teens experience, plus the baggage of an overpharmaceuticalized worldview. Many do and will eventually challenge that view, but in the meantime, life is increasingly colored by their early pharma identity.

Consider college, a time when young adults take on all kinds of important personal challenges. For twenty-seven years, Gertrude Carter helped them do just that. Carter, a self-described "old-school" brand of counselor and the director of psychological services at Bennington College in Vermont is a widely admired observer of psychological trends in university life, about which she has a wry sense of humor and sharp analytical views. (Of the difference between Bennington and Williams College students, she once said that "Bennington tends to be more bulimic — or defiant — whereas Williams tends to be more anorexic — or compliant.") Her therapeutic métier is one-on-one counseling. Working at the college for so long, she has witnessed a consistent percentage of students coming in for psychological help; every school year for more than two decades, about 30 percent of Bennington students would go to the counseling center for help with everything from loneliness to heartbreak to despair to problems with alcohol and drugs. "The percent of students seeking help hasn't changed at all," she says. "Neither has the seriousness of their problems."

But beginning in 1995, something big did change. The percentage of students coming in for help who were already on Ritalin, Prozac, and other psych meds rose from about 5 percent to about 45 percent. At college campuses nationally, the trend was less dramatic but still clear: the portion of students who went to health centers who were already taking psych meds went from 7 percent in 1992 to 18 percent in 2000. And they wanted to stay on the drugs. Carter didn't object to the meds per se, but to the poor medical practices that usually surrounded and fed their use by students. Typically, a student would come for help and ask for a new prescription for a drug he or she had been on for years. The center's physician would request the student's medical histories — standard procedure in establishing a new physician-patient relationship. "Those records are typically horrendous," Carter has said. In them she usually found few diagnostic, psychosocial, or psychiatric evaluations, the core of almost all therapeutic protocols for psychiatric meds. She also found few if any ongoing treatment plans either, and that burned her up.

Writing in the *Chronicle of Higher Education* with Dr. Jeffrey Winseman, a psychiatrist she hired to handle the center's growing pharma load, Carter let the fur fly: "These fractured interactions with caregivers seem to mirror the child's past inconsistent interactions with [previous physicians]. [The students'] need to restore and strengthen interpersonal relationships is not recognized in the effort to control symptoms with medication. The message is, *'If you are to remain stable emotionally and attain academic success, stay on medications to handle all problems.'*" Of course, the pair also noted, that was not surprising, particularly given the economic imperative: "Kaiser Permanente, one of the first HMOs, recently published guidelines for the treatment of depression which suggested that psychotherapy be recommended only after two consecutive trials of antidepressant medication have failed."

To get a better handle on the issue, particularly Ritalin use, Carter and Winseman requested that Novartis send a representative to discuss the uses of their drug and, just as important, a way to track the growing abuse of Ritalin on campus. Ritalin is, after

all, a class II controlled substance, and several prominent researchers have over recent years raised concerns that it might be
a classic "gateway" drug, opening the door to abuse of other substances. (Ritalin trading is rampant at select high schools.) They
heard nothing. The pair continued to call the company. Eventually Novartis informed them that it had decided "not to promote Ritalin." This was interesting — OK, it was a stretch —
given that the company was then preparing the launch of two
new Ritalin-based products. "I never understood why they could
not send a rep. They seem so eager ordinarily," Carter says.

To Carter and Winseman, one of the most important ramifi-
cations of the counseling to medication-only shift was how it
might alter the overall development of young people. "Students
who request medicine for their problems . . . often discount their
own ability to begin to modulate the rhythms of their lives,"
they worried. The medication-only approach "does not encourage self-reflection or responsible self-regulation. A medication-
only approach fails to encourage the hallmark of late adolescent
development, the dramatic increase in capacity for self-examina-
tion and ability to think critically, the development of responsibility for one's self."

There were, to be sure, more than a few defenders of the meds.
Ed Weismeier, the head of student health at UCLA, saw SSRIs
as a huge boost for troubled students, particularly those over-
whelmed by the scale and intensity of big campus life. Weismeier was a pragmatist. "There are more young people who can
succeed in a university environment because of the drugs who
could not have twenty years ago," he says. "The drugs allow
them to succeed . . . and most respond reasonably well to the
SSRIs without a lot of counseling visits."

But what else was happening to them as a result? Gary
Margolis, the director of counseling at Middlebury College in
Vermont, reported that "the old relationship of mutual communication has transformed into 'What can you give me to feel
better and perform?' I say this descriptively, not pejoratively.
They have seen the Pac-Man version of neurotransmitter theory
and they come in quoting it." And, more troubling, "Students are
sharing the drugs," Margolis says, "particularly at the end of the

semester, and also, frankly, there is a party use of the drugs — so you can perform well at a party!"

There was a new wave of pharmaceutical populism — a growing campus culture of self-diagnosis and self-prescription. In the freshman dormitory at one private college in Los Angeles, it is now common, particularly among female students, simply to skip the counseling office altogether and instead rely on a tight-knit network of prescription drug users, some of whom are very well informed. "I didn't take any prescription drugs when I got here, but my roommate, who is depressed and bulimic, did. She was so out of control but wouldn't go to the counseling center for help," one student, who asked to remain anonymous, confided in an interview. "So, basically, I became the mother. I read up on the drugs and called her on her bullshit when she wasn't taking them the right way. And that got around and before I knew it I became 'the Prozac mom' for the whole floor [of the dorm]. I can tell you which drugs go with which other ones. I know how to get somebody off Paxil [which has a severe withdrawal syndrome]. I even tried it myself for a while."

But were the drugs really working? If pills sans counseling was now, practically speaking, the treatment of choice, how could you tell if the patient was getting better? Norman Hoffman, the head of Student Mental Health Services at McGill University in Montreal, started asking that question when he noticed more and more students, especially those from the United States, taking what was known as "the California cocktail: Neurontin (the anti-epileptic prescribed off label for, among other things, bipolar disorder), Wellbutrin (an antidepressant from Glaxo), and Ritalin." Typically, he says, students will report that, since taking the drugs, they are "better." But when he looked at the student more closely, he says, "They are not 'better.' Their grades are not better, and if you can get them to stick around for six months or so, you begin to find out the whole picture: they don't sleep well, they are drinking, they are procrastinating and not eating right. They soon find out that they have outgrown the biological [need] for the drug that they may genuinely have had as a child."

There looms in all of this, to be sure, more than a hint of generational politics. Dr. Richard Keeling, a former president of the American College Health Association and perhaps the dean of those who study student drug use patterns, recalls that, "Back in 1993, [counseling centers] were still running on issues like gender identity and the struggle with it, but over the years we noticed a big drop-off in the number of students coming into the center. We assumed we were doing something wrong and changed our hours and approach, but there was still no change. We finally saw that it was not us . . . Pills to them are just part of what people do. There is no stigma."

That there is no stigma attached to the act of seeking help for mental health problems is clearly a positive development. But what of Gen-Rx1's impulse to accept drugs as the first resort? There are signs that the industry's educational efforts are registering at a younger and younger age. In a symposium entitled "Development of School-based Adolescent Depression Awareness Program," presented at the annual convention of the American Psychiatric Association, researchers noted two trends in "depression literacy" among kids and educators. One was that there was an increase in the number of kids who said "no" when asked if they agreed with the statement "Medicine should not be used to treat mental illness." The other was the growing belief among teachers of health classes that "getting depression out of the coping skills section of health ed and into the illness section" was a priority. The intent was to underscore the seriousness of depression; arguably, the effect was to make it completely the province of medicine, and, by extension, of pharma.

Today, the focus on prescription drugs for children transcends psych meds. Across the board, pharmaceutical companies are investing unprecedented sums in clinical trials of drugs for young people — by last count some 194 different compounds. Many of these trials are long-awaited and needed and will give physicians a better handle on how the young metabolize drugs differently from adults. Many are for medications that target chronic conditions that will require lifelong dosing. As Dr. Richard Gorman, chair of the Committee on Drugs of the American Academy of Pediatrics, commented in a 2002 article in the *New England*

Journal of Medicine: "We are entering what could be the golden age for kids and pharmaceuticals."

GEN-RX2: THE MIDDLE-YEARS TRIBE

In the great scrum of middle age, we all dodge the body blocks as best we can. The advice on how to do so seems to come so fast, and with such authority: we should be concerned about cholesterol, we should watch our blood pressure, our blood sugar, our weight, our diet. If we don't, we're screwed. On any given day, one can be driven crazy about another new thing that can go horribly wrong. As we are only human, we consciously or unconsciously pick from this vast field our major health battles. The rest we hope to hold at bay by any convenient means possible. We are a tribe of conscious risk dodgers. As such, we are perhaps the most agile of the new pharma tribes. Risk management is our birthright.

The best evidence of that is in the growing generational consensus about cholesterol and high blood pressure, and the pills we take to control those conditions. Statins, designed to lower bad cholesterol, seem to work. Ditto ACE inhibitors, designed to combat hypertension, albeit only, as it turns out, after first trying the much less expensive (and off-patent) diuretics. Whether the drugs actually reduce overall deaths from heart disease is still hotly debated. But the collective scientific opinion about statins and hypertension drugs is growing so quickly that it is only a matter of time before they are prescribed for almost everyone over fifty. Already there is a pill, Caduet by Pfizer, that combines cholesterol and blood pressure drugs. We buy the rationale for such drugs as a culture. They are our flak jackets.

Yet the critic may well say that such drugs encourage imprudent lifestyle choices — why modify our diet and get more exercise if we can do it with a pill and thus get more time to work or watch TV? But that line of reasoning does a fast dance around two important facts: many people cannot control their cholesterol or blood pressure with lifestyle changes alone, and a physician cannot withhold treatment just because a patient is non-compliant. These facts of medical life are routinely exploited by the industry. (A recent advertisement for Crestor, a new statin yet to fulfill its original sales ambition, is framed, in full color, by a cornucopia of fresh vegetables.) Does that mean many of the "wrong" people are taking statins? Perhaps. But there is also evidence that not enough of the "right" people are on them, particularly the poor.

Yet members of the statin-ACE tribe do share the winking notion that they have put fate on hold. Daily pills have become a reminder of risk, consciously reduced. It is a tribe that is constantly being expanded by pharma, its belief systems reinforced by some of the most sophisticated software programs in the world.

Not all of Gen-Rx2 resides in risk-management land. The tribe divides and then subdivides again. Not surprisingly for a generation that works more than one hundred hours a year more than its elders, many members are concerned with performance and productivity, and with drugs that can either heighten and sustain that, or counteract the problems that come from being too productive too much of the time.

The most noted new subtribe is adults with attention deficit disorder. Like ADD in children, ADD in adults can be a truly disabling condition. Until recently it was rarely diagnosed because it was long believed that ADD subsided in adulthood. Later research showed that only the hyperactivity component of ADD receded; the lack of focus continued. Researchers knew this for years, but ADD in adults was still underdiagnosed. What changed all of that was work, specifically the demands of the modern workplace. Once a place of relative predictability, work in the late 1990s was actually celebrated for its fractiousness and unpredictability; that is what allegedly makes work so "creative" and "fulfilling." It is what makes companies innovative and profitable, and ever demanding of increased productivity.

But such traits are also what made a new group of ADD sufferers finally take action — that, and a huge new spending campaign by Novartis and others to redefine the tribe. Perhaps the most important permutation was the popularization of a new tribal belief: that ADD was a playpen-to-grave disorder. In a media alert at the 2003 convention of the American Psychiatric Association, the public relations firm Fleishman-Hillard, hired by McNeil Pharmaceuticals, set down the new touchstone: "What do D's in school, increased risk of driving accidents, substance abuse, and jumping from job to job have in common? All could be the serious consequences of not managing and treating ADHD in all life stages." The answer was Concerta, McNeil's new once-a-day compound for the disorder. Lilly, too, had its own entrant into the adult ADD field. As one Lilly researcher explained to an APA audience, "Continuous symptom relief is the key message. 'In the evening and into the morning.' That reaches families where they live — it's not just about getting through the school day."

Where the old ADD pitch had once been about behavior and performance, now the tribal custodians, from CHADD to the APA, began to introduce the notion of job productivity as a barometer of the disorder and its treatment. An article in *Attention!*, CHADD's member magazine, summed it up. One way to achieve a goal of treatment was by "outlining your map to productivity." It was good advice. But it was also identical to that found in countless self-improvement books for people without ADD: find a way to organize tasks visually, avoid making lists that are too long and thus overwhelming, use your PC to write goal and task outlines, and invest in a personal digital assistant to make sure that you follow through. The author then listed a number of Web links for the adult ADD sufferer. They were almost all work-related, ranging from Lotus.com, the software giant, to Inspiration.com, which is a "graphical outliner that enables users to flip back and forth between a flow chart and an outline." To drive home the urgency of the disorder to physicians, companies like McNeil came up with ways to sensitize reluctant prescribers. One, on display and in almost constant use at the APA convention, was a combination of high-tech goggles that showed how difficult it was to read and organize information from the point of view of an adult with ADHD. It was, literally, a simpatico headset.

At the 2003 APA convention, a new diagnostic tool emerged. It was not a test so much as it was a series of "profiles" of the adult ADD sufferer who might benefit from pharmacology. As Dr. Calvin Sumner, an ADD expert who just happened to be hovering near the Concerta exhibit explained, "ADHD is not a disease, it's an organizational disorder. But it's not about 'getting your act together.'" Then what is it about? "What's working is putting clear boundaries around what it is, how it manifests. It's identifying the habits of [people's] lives that can be treated. For example, there is the woman who needs twenty hours to prepare for a brief instead of five." That was one profile of a person who could benefit from treatment. "Or the person who seems to have all the right stuff for a promotion, who is just on the edge of getting that big raise, and then, time and time again, blows it by doing something like showing up late to a meeting with the president of the company." That was another. "So part of our job is now to put a face on the disorder."

The ideology of the tribe got tweaked as well. In the past, one of the most important ADD credos, at least in terms of its ability to destigmatize the condition and ease the pressure on parents, was about variances in glucose metabolism in some areas of the brain. Now the belief system shifted. Changes in "executive function" — the ability to focus and organize information governed by the prefrontal lobe — became the new credo. As did the role of genes. "Of particular interest to researchers studying the heritability of the disorder are the d-4 dopamine receptor and dopamine transporter genes," an article on adult ADD in *Attention!* noted. "Both play a role in the functioning of the frontal lobe . . . the secretary of the brain."

Of course, all tribes change. It is how they survive. For medical tribes, the introduction of new science information is a good thing. But when a medical tribe is largely driven by pharma, as in the case of ADD, something else is going on as well. Appetite for product is expanded. Focus gets shifted from the environment, in this case the workplace, to the individual. Consider: Whereas there were few adults taking ADD drugs as recently as five years ago, there are now tens of thousands of adult users of Ritalin and the like. And they will be taking it for the rest of their lives, at least if they follow the latest tribal dictates.

Two of the hottest drugs for the middle-aged treat two states of being: sleep and waking. They are both sold and taken based on anxiety about productivity. In the realm of sleep, pharma has historically struggled. A pill to make one nod off, at will, was long a quest not unlike that of an anti-fat pill, and like that effort it was fraught with peril. Most discoveries to induce sleep simply did not work well, or had huge abuse potential. In the late 1980s, Halcion became a standard business traveler's drug for insomnia, and it was prescribed on a dime. Then it fell from grace because of horrific side effects that its maker had not adequately addressed: it made a small percentage of takers violent and hostile. Doctors grew wary of prescribing for insomnia, and the condition fell from the list of hot chronic conditions.

Then, in 1993, the French company Sanofi-Synthelab had a breakthrough with a drug it called Ambien. The drug acted on the GABA complex of neurotransmitters, which promote sleep by stopping brain cells from firing. Ambien made a person sleep pretty well and did not seem to cause day-after sluggishness. Using statistics from the nonprofit National Sleep Foundation (NSF), Sanofi was able to make a convincing case that insomnia was an undertreated condition, with only about 40 percent of all sufferers getting help. Ambien won FDA approval. A big part of its subsequent marketing campaign focused on how sleep deprivation costs the economy $45 billion a year in lost productivity, health care, and accident-related expenses. "Half of all office workers sleep poorly at least a few times a week," the NSF announced, "and 65 percent say they have trouble concentrating because of it." The company then initiated a huge DTC sleep awareness campaign, focusing on the long-term dangers of not getting enough quality rest — how lack of sleep led to impaired insulin secretion and a drop in the body's ability to fight infection, as well as car crashes and, for women, a higher risk of developing heart disease. The campaign paid off, and Ambien became a blockbuster.

But what if sleep was not the problem, or not perceived as a problem? What if a person was simply sluggish on the job and wanted to feel better? In the late 1990s, in patient surveys, staying *awake* was the issue about which most people complained. The middle-years tribe demanded: How about something to keep me going? Again, pharma had historic problems selling "wakefulness" drugs. They were stimulants, yet stimulants were a double-edged sword, with huge sales potential but equally huge side effects and abuse problems. There was another problem: you could not get the FDA to approve a drug for treating "decreased productivity." Not yet.

The solution, for a company named Cephalon, was a stimulant compound named modafinil, branded as Provigil. The drug was, by comparison to its chemical siblings, a fairly mild stimulant, and studies showed that it had a benign side-effect profile. It was clean, if a drug can ever be such a thing. In 1998 Cephalon won FDA approval to market Provigil for the only thing it seemed fit for — as a treatment for severe narcolepsy, a serious disorder that often causes patients to drop off into deep sleep, quickly and without any warning. Almost immediately the company ran into problems. There were only about 50,000 diagnosed narcoleptics in the whole country, and just getting them to the physician to ask for treatment was problematic. Many people with narcolepsy simply accepted it as their fate, or viewed the condition, as did their employers, as indicative of laziness. Their physicians were still leery of stimulants. In short, there was no tribal thinking about insufficient wakefulness — yet.

To build a more receptive audience, Cephalon mounted a big awareness campaign. The core of it was that excessive sleepiness — for that, technically, was one way to enlarge the more restrictive label of narcolepsy — is a serious medical problem. It had nothing to do with laziness, and it could be a health threat. Not only could it lead to fatal accidents, but it was hard on the body in many other ways. The most compelling argument for Provigil was fundamentally tied up with work. Excessive sleepiness, for whatever reason, led to an increase in the "error rate." As one of Cephalon's physician–thought leaders later explained to the *New York Times:* "In terms of error rate, 18 hours of no sleep, which is what many of us regularly do, is equivalent to a blood alcohol level of .05. Twenty-one hours of no sleep is equivalent to a blood alcohol level of .08, which is illegal in many states." Excessive sleepiness . . . was illegal!

Cephalon then asked the FDA to expand Provigil's indication to include all forms of abnormal sleepiness. The agency turned down the request, but approved another indication, "work shift sleep disorder" — which essentially meant all truckers, medical interns, and software programmers under thirty. Once that message was out, the excessively sleepy began coming out of the proverbial woodwork. To make it easier to ask for a prescription and get it, Cephalon set up a Web site, which gave potential patients a short test rating their propensity to fall asleep while doing things like watching TV, "lying down to rest in the afternoon," or "sitting quietly after lunch (when you've had no alcohol)." If they scored more than a 10 (as I did in spades), they were to take the test to their physician, for whom the site offered a "reimbursement assistance hotline."

Sales exploded. By 2003, worldwide sales of Provigil hit $290 million, on its way to an estimated $400 million by the end of 2004. Some 60 percent of those sales came from patients in the United States. Something else: it was almost all (90 percent) prescribed off label. That is, doctors, seeing that the drug had few safety problems, were willing to prescribe Provigil even if someone did not have classic narcolepsy, or even classic work shift sleep disorder. The popularization of excessive sleepiness as a risk factor had trumped that. After all, who among us who works *doesn't* have work shift sleepiness? A "shift" is in the eye — and body — of the beholder. As Mark Goodman, a pharmaceuticals analyst at Morgan Stanley, commented, "No one would ever have believed it would be this big. Everyone viewed narcolepsy as the market and did not appreciate the benign side-effect profile and how that would play into off-label use." Even college students began to use the drug, which prompted Cephalon to look at using Provigil for childhood ADD.

In the celebration of wakefulness that followed, there were, of course, the usual Crabby Appletons who complained that dosing people for what was essentially everyday sleepiness was a bad thing, that it increased the possibility that people would use the drug as a way to skimp on sleep intentionally, which, as Sanofi was busy telling people in its Ambien campaign, weakens the immune system. "The drug enables us to be that much more workaholic and that much more obsessed with accomplishments and productivity, and I think our society is already extreme along those lines," Dr. Martha J. Farah, director of the Center for Cognitive Neuroscience at the University of Pennsylvania, told the *New York Times* in the summer of 2004. "The natural checks on that tendency, like needing to go to bed, are being rolled back by modafinil." But by then, the wakefulness party was on.

Risk management, performance, productivity — all perfect tribes for a work-based culture. But work, to amend William James, is a bitch-goddess, and humans can take only so much before they begin to seek comfort from its excess. You can smoke and you can drink or you can gamble or you can porn out, and that will take the edge off, for a while. Or, you could use your growing pharmaceutical literacy to get comfort another way — through opiates and opioids.

That was the line I heard in the late 1990s, when a friend of mine, an executive at one of the major studios, began telling me about something called "Vicodin Fridays." Every Friday, one executive would make the rounds of his colleagues' offices, bearing a handful of white, capsule-shaped tablets. The tablets were Vicodin, the brand name for a powerful synthetic opioid named hydrocodone, available by prescription only. It was a painkiller, but that was not why these men and women took it. They took it, as my friend told me, to "numb out," after a week of constant work pressure. When they went home for the weekend, carrying the requisite ten scripts that had to be read by Monday morning, they had an additional stash. They called what they did "taking a Vicodin weekend."

All right, there has always been drug abuse in the entertainment business. *Quelle horreur!* Rebellion, via drug use, is sexy and salable. And fast money breeds fast times. But this was different. There was no fun in Vicodin Fridays, no rebellion or even any major highly cool posing. The pills had simply become part of work. Because the executives were rich, the pills were easy for them to obtain. They just sent their people to fetch, as did their ideological opposite, Rush Limbaugh, who announced his opioid addiction in 2003. (He also proved that, his own antidrug crusading messages to the contrary, you can indeed "work high.")

Yet it wasn't just the elite. In the late 1990s, off-label opioid use for pure vocational relaxation seemed, suddenly, to be all around. And it was a middle- to upper-middle-class phenomenon.

Why were the drugs so easy to get? A big reason was physician laziness and overwork. Vicodin and its molecular sisters were one way to control acute and chronic pain, without repeat office visits. The other reason was prescriber licentiousness. Beginning in the early 1990s, physicians were pressed by a number of pain-patient organizations, some with educational grants from major opioid makers, to prescribe opioids for deep, persistent pain. The cause was a righteous one: traditionally, American doctors had underprescribed the drugs to legitimate pain sufferers. Yet soon pain was recognized as a "fifth vital sign." State legislatures passed a number of what became known as "intractable pain laws," which spelled out the physicians' pain-relief obligations. The result was a frenzy of script writing. And abuse. According to one government study, the number of first-time abusers of opioids grew from about 500,000 initiates annually in 1989 to more than 1.6 million in 1998. By 2002, mentions of Vicodin by emergency room staff — a key barometer of abuse — had risen 170 percent over 1994, from 9,300 to 25,000.

It was an amazing phenomenon, mainly for how little it was noted. Most of the press about opioid abuse centered not on the middle class to well-off, but on the poor and the rural — losers and hicks scoring the more powerful OxyContin, a.k.a. "hillbilly heroin" — in places like Kentucky and West Virginia. Yet the real action (and perhaps the more relevant as a portal to the future) was in the suburbs, because it was there that opioid abuse was soaring — and doing so, at least ostensibly, because people knew how to get it. They didn't have to knock off a drugstore; they just used their telephone and a Blue Cross card.

For physicians and psychiatrists who treated addiction, the change of clientele was palpable. "What we are seeing now are bright, aggressive people — some at the crest of careers — who may start out on the drug for, say, a weekend sprained ankle, then find out how great it feels to be on it," says Dr. Clifford Bernstein, a pain and addiction specialist at the Waismann Institute, one of several nationwide centers that advertise "Vicodin detox" right alongside heroin, morphine, and cocaine detox. "Eventually they find that Vicodin rounds out the corners of life. Some of them actually think they deserve it and are ingenious at finding ways to get it." In the parlance of self-help, they know how to find the cheese. As David Crausman, a Los Angeles psychologist who treats many such boomer dopers, notes: "All of the attributes of the winner in today's economy — agility, problem solving, learning a system and knowing how to work it — that's exactly what addicts need to do. They've read the *PDR* [*Physicians' Desk Reference*]! They've read the medical journals. They even know the side effects, so they can tell you, for example, that they are on certain other drugs that preclude you from prescribing a non-opioid."

There were other signs of creative self-prescribing as well. One concerned pet allergies. Many people who suffered from Fido's fur didn't bother with a prescription for Claritin (60 percent of which was consumed by patients without diagnosed allergies). They simply went out and bought some Pepcid, an over-the-counter heartburn drug that was discovered — no one knew by whom — to alleviate sneezing and sniffling among those with pet allergies. What would be the physical cost if one used it too often for that purpose? Again, no one knew, but it didn't seem to matter.

This suburban drug sprawl marked the same kind of pharmaceutical populism that was going on in college dorms. If you knew what "worked," why engage a doctor's advice? Who cared about the intent of the drug? Just get the pills. It is an attitude that has exploded with the onslaught of Internet prescription drug sites; one can buy almost anything with minimal physician involvement.

And how different was that from what pharma itself had been doing with heartburn and GERD and its popular treatments? By 2004, the ad campaign for Tagamet, now available over the counter, was literally in the neighborhood bar and fast food joint. To heck with GERD, Glaxo now proclaimed, Tagamet could help you indulge yourself. Where it once was sold as a treatment for unintentional excess, it now was sold for intentional partying. In taverns, Glaxo circulated coasters and glasses emblazoned with provocative young women in tight shirts, asking, "Did you bring protection?" The company targeted Atlanta because of its population's consumption of spicy food. As the creator of the campaign put it, "A lot of younger people aren't really interested in being told they're going to suffer a lot. We're telling them that they're probably living a pretty good lifestyle and probably want to continue leading that lifestyle."

After all, how different was self-prescription from what was happening at physicians' offices, where off-label prescribing was rampant? Was it really so surprising that "what works now" should become the dominant force in prescribing drugs, rather than "what is proven safe and effective"?

Whatever the answer, one thing was clear for Gen-Rx2: a new prescription culture — expanded, self-justifying, increasingly outside the domain of the physician — was exploding inside and outside their own office doors.

GEN-RX3: SUPERSENIORS AND THE TRIBE OF HIGH-PERFORMANCE AGING

Seniors, the elderly, the aged — whatever term one might want to use in describing those over the arbitrary age line of sixty-five — have always been big consumers of pharmaceuticals. And why not? That we want ourselves or our parents to live longer, better, and more comfortable lives is utterly human; that we do everything we can to do so is utterly understandable. And so it is no surprise that the most popular prescription drugs for seniors are drugs that also occupy the handiest shelf for the middle-aged tribe. Their position there represents a triumph of pharma's theology of long-term, continuous treatment for lifelong chronic conditions. There — right up on *Modern Maturity*'s list of top sellers (as of 2003) — are statins for cholesterol control, COX-2 inhibitors for pain, proton pump inhibitors for GERD, beta-blockers and ACE inhibitors for high blood pressure, SSRIs for depression. Save for one category of disease treatment — osteoporosis — they are all drugs that take root in the middle years.

On top of that list, however, is another list of drugs specifically designed to treat the diseases most associated with aging, the so-called gray illnesses: Alzheimer's (affecting about 4 million seniors), geriatric depression (2 million), diabetes (6.3 million), osteoarthritis (20 million), osteoporosis (10 million), Parkinson's (1.5 million), prostate disorders (about half of all sixty-plus males), and rheumatoid arthritis (2.1 million). Over the past decade, pharma has responded forcefully to this market, developing 200 new medications. Another 150 are currently under development. The meta-result: 75 percent of all those over sixty-five years of age now take prescription medications on a daily basis, with most of them averaging between two and four different prescriptions a day. Polypharmacy has become the norm.

In long-term-care homes, pharmaceuticals are overwhelmingly used for behavioral management. About 58 percent of residents are on some form of psych medication, a huge increase over the past decade despite growing restrictions on seniors' use of these drugs. Among the most popular are antipsychotics, antianxiety agents, and hypnotics — all used for behavior management. Then there are the antidepressants, prescribed to about one third of all residents who take psych meds. Much of this pattern grows out of pharma's new sales push at such institutions; the number of sales contacts at chronic-care facilities grew by 8 percent in 2002 alone.

In the general senior population, the two biggest pharma tribes for chronic disease are those concerned with diabetes, and those concerned with osteoarthritis and osteoporosis.

In the best case, today's "gray diabetics" rarely resemble their predecessors. In many ways, they are better off: new, easier ways of testing blood sugar are widely available and often reimbursed by the chintziest of health plans. That is important, because tight control of blood sugar is the centerpiece of all diabetes treatment, whether involving drugs or not. New drugs are constantly being developed as well, and with them new disease management plans, often developed by pharma and offered for free. Diabetes now drives all kinds of business and cultural change. In inner-city drugstores, it is now common to find entire diabetes care sections, and special waiting areas for customers seeking diabetes counseling from pharmacy staff. There are specialized pharma detailing initiatives in Spanish, Chinese, and Korean. The disease is so widespread — affecting about 18 percent of all in the sixty-five-plus group — and awareness is so high that the modern senior often finds himself being detailed in an ever widening "diabetes world," even if he is not diabetic.

Osteoarthritis, the kind many of us will experience to one degree or another, is also rampant. Here the pharma presence is huge, driven in large part by two companies, Merck and Pfizer, whose respective blockbusters, Vioxx (at least until it was withdrawn in late 2004) and Celebrex, have fueled a new recognition of the disease. Today there are entire magazines dedicated to the condition, shelves of books about treating and preventing it. They are almost all underwritten by pharmaceutical companies, some more so than others.

But the pharma-senior link that underwent the biggest transformation over the past decade involves osteoporosis, the natural weakening of the human bone as one ages. For decades, pharma's main connection to the condition was ancillary, through its promotion of hormone replacement therapy (HRT) to menopausal women, which was mainly prescribed and consumed because it alleviated the sometimes unbearable effects of menopause. Then, in the mid-1990s, the ancillary became the primary. Part of the reason was damage control: increasingly, HRT was suspected of a wide range of serious adverse effects, including increased risk of stroke, heart disease, and cancer. More important, studies showed that, of all those sixty-five or older who fell and fractured a hip, 20 percent would die within a year of the fall. Few studies showed how often, in reality, seniors fell. But with the population aging, there was suddenly an urgent market for a drug that "cured" osteoporosis. Merck and Lilly responded with major new drug development programs.

Just as important was the creation of a test that would justify the prescribing of a drug that reduced risk of fracture — a way to create a tribe. This every major drug company did by backing the use of bone mineral density testing, or BMD. BMD was and is controversial. While it is associated with fracture, "It is not a sufficiently accurate predictor of individual's risk of fracture to be used as a guide to therapy," as one recent article in the *British Medical Journal* put it. But of all the risk signals of osteoporosis — sedentary lifestyle, poor nutrition, insufficient calcium intake, overuse of alcohol — BMD could be measured easily and scientifically. Pharma poured millions into a campaign to establish it as the universal measurement for fracture risk, including the sponsorship of the World Health Organization subcommittee that made the most important recommendations for BMD use. The strategy worked. With pharma's encouragement, the National Osteoarthritis Foundation publicized a central recommendation based on the WHO finding: all women over the age of sixty-five should have a BMD. The organization also articulated a cohesive new belief system: Osteoporosis was not an "inevitable" part of aging; it could be arrested with the right combination of drugs and lifestyle. If it were not, the disease could be fatal. The result was a flourishing of osteoporosis as a serious diagnosis for seniors, and a blossoming of sales for Lilly's Evista and Merck's Fosamax.

But pharma's experience with osteoporosis did more than merely create a new tribe. It opened up pharma to a grand new vision of its role in the life of the average senior. The undisputed prophet of that tribe is Sid Taurel, the chairman and CEO of Eli Lilly, and, not incidentally, the chairman of the National Osteoporosis Foundation's annual fundraising event, the Silhouette Ball.

Taurel, born in Morocco and schooled in France, is the ulti-

mate one-company man in a world of shifting, ever jumping alliances and chairmanships. He has spent almost all of his professional life at Lilly. As such, he has a rare command of the
company's specifics and culture. Intense but mild-mannered, elegant, intellectually agile, and a little world-weary, Taurel has
long occupied the topmost rungs of pharma high-wire acts. He is
responsible for building the world's largest factory for the production of drugs for diabetes, and he is a consummate defender
of Lilly's burgeoning business in psychiatric drugs, Prozac chief
among them. He is capable of umbrage, a refreshing characteristic in a world of bland. Once, when I asked him if Lilly's constant
bombardment of ads about depression didn't constitute, in effect, the "medicalization of everyday life," Taurel looked visibly
hurt. Then he lectured: "I cannot agree with that at all. We are
helping identify diseases that are there and are not being diagnosed or treated. We are not creating disease. That criticism may
come from slippages in the use of drugs beyond their [approved]
indications. But that is because there are genuine gray areas in
the diagnosis of mental conditions . . . But we do not create disease!"

In recent years, Taurel has taken to the stump to promote what
he regards as "the dominant public policy issue of the first half
of the new century: [that] the future of America is inextricably
bound with the future of aging and the progress of biomedicine."
At the center of Taurel's crusade stands a well-established observation: by 2030, more than 20 percent of the U.S. population will
be sixty-five or older, a stunning number given that only 13 percent are that age today. More: as a nation, we are living longer
than ever before, and, as Taurel pointed out at a recent Town
Hall meeting in Los Angeles, we are living *longer and healthier*.
He likes to cite data collected since the early 1980s that show
that disability among the aged is steadily dropping. Disability
dropped 1.6 percent annually from 1989 through 1994, and 2.6
percent per year from 1994 through 1999. "Today," he says, "less
then nineteen percent of Americans over sixty-five suffer from a
disabling condition." And that, he says, is a direct result of two
things: improvements in lifestyles and improvements in medi

cine. "This longer health span created by medical innovations may turn out to be one of the nation's most precious natural resources."

But Taurel isn't content merely to state the record. As he and numerous pharma executives now see it, the aged of today and the near future represent a profound, world-changing shift in the way we live. "Retirees today are not buying rocking chairs," Taurel told the Town Hall audience. "They are buying sea kayaks and tandem bikes. They are taking up distance running in their sixties, learning to tap-dance in their seventies, and signing up for walking tours at eighty." It all added up to "the emergence of a new life stage — growing between what we have always called middle age, say age fifty, and what we think of as truly old age, a boundary that has now moved out to seventy-five or eighty. It's as if we've opened the circle of life and inserted a new wedge in it . . . The people entering this new age will not turn into their grandparents. Instead, they are turning out to be simply more experienced versions of themselves in middle age." Seventy was the new forty.

I asked Taurel what, exactly, was Lilly's biggest contribution to this new health span. "Basically, we are building new bone," he said. "Our drugs for osteoporosis are at the forefront of doing that, and their use is just one more indication of how my generation has always grabbed hold of its destiny from day one."

The supersenior message has been taken up widely. Arguably one of the hottest publishing phenomena in health titles is something that might be called "RX-plus." In RX-plus books, mainstream physicians do what non-mainstream "health experts" used to do: give advice about how to live longer. The books often combine advice for using approved medications in combination with special diets, vitamins, exercise regimens, and nontraditional practices like yoga and meditation. Such was the approach of Dr. Bob Arnot's *Breast Cancer Prevention Diet*, which argued for the use of flaxseed oil in tandem with traditional medicine, and Drs. William Shankle and Daniel Amen's *Preventing Alzheimer's*, which combines traditional pharma meds with such things as "mental exercise," omega-3 fatty acids, red rice yeast extract, and coenzyme Q, to delay or prevent the diseases.

The king of the RX-plus genre is Dr. Steven Lamm, an internist and clinical assistant professor at New York University School of Medicine. "Staying young is the new American dream," he writes. "Men and women are keenly aware that in a world where fatigue is the enemy, faltering memory a disaster zone, and illness a pitfall to be avoided, keeping their mental and physical edges razor-sharp is the only way to sustain and live a full life. Today, it's actually possible to lower age barriers, make our minds and bodies even better, and maintain that hard-won competitive edge through a combination of breakthrough medical discoveries and the aggressive use of what I call Vitality Medicine."

In book after book, Lamm, who describes himself as a "Pfizer Professor" (he has won one of the company's research awards), has taken on every aspect of life, from weight problems (*Thinner at Last*), to erectile dysfunction (*The Virility Solution*), to aging (*Younger at Last*). The key to his approach lies in finding the "right" physician, one who will be willing to prescribe the off-label treatments Lamm recommends in his Vitality Medicine armamentarium. "In your search," he writes in *Younger at Last*, "you are going to come across physicians who may initially be skeptical of any medication, technique, or new technology that has not already been proven to be successful with an indisputable double-blind study. This would not be the right physician for you. The very essence of Vitality Medicine has to do with flexibility, change, and a willingness to 'experiment.'" Among some of his techniques: nitroglycerin cream for erection enhancement, testosterone to up sexual drive, deprenyl (usually used for Parkinson's) to enhance female libido, trazodone (an older antidepressant) to banish sexual exhaustion, "sensual touch" (because it releases the hormone oxytocin) to alleviate sexual tension, endermology (the use of a machine that sucks the skin) to get rid of cellulite, and, of course, laser resurfacing and antioxidants.

Lamm's experimental ethos may not be for everyone. His newest book, *The Virility Solution*, named the impotence drug, Vasomax, as "fast-acting with virtually no side effects" — despite the fact that, upon publication, Vasomax hasn't even been submitted to the FDA for review. But that does not mean that Lamm is a quack — it just means that he, like so many other physicians in both the clinic and the classroom, are inclined to follow pharma's cultural and experimental lead.

In the timeline of Generation Rx, all of these trends started to add up. By the early years of the millennium, one could begin to see a line between senior traditionalists — people who sought medical treatment to cure traditional medical complaints — and superseniors — men and women who bought the notion that they did not have to be their grandparents. The medical culture morphed over and over again, and while pharma set the dominant tone, it was not always in control, particularly among seniors, who had had a lifetime of dealing with the industry as the background noise to their medical decisions.

Outside the traditional medical establishment, the supersenior mindset spiraled onward and upward. There were new medical associations dedicated to nothing else but the notion that aging could be reversed. (If one were a think-tanker, one might even say that a whole new psychographic was being conceived.) For those who could afford it, there were specialized medical resorts, with specialized medico-spa treatments. Many, like Las Vegas's Cenegenics Medical Institute, which the *Wall Street Journal* described as a sprawling neoclassical spa that resembles the White House, combine the spa feel with injections of human growth hormone. It is a big business, with about 35 percent of the center's 4,000 patients getting daily injections of HGH for everything from increased libido to decreased wrinkles. And that does not include the vitamins and testosterone. Rock on . . .

By the turn of this century, superseniorism, like risk reduction and performance drugs, was doing one thing above all else: it was creating and expanding a new pharmaceutical appetite — and among seniors, the appetite for pills, by the end of the 1990s, seemed to know no end. Putting aside all of the off-label prescribing and the taking of supplements, seniors were using more pills than ever before. Over-the-counter medication use was also at an all-time high. Among seniors and, for that matter, the general population, polypharmacy was no longer seen as a problem. It was an opportunity.

And it was, when one backed up and looked at it all — away from the political Sturm und Drang of Medicare drug benefits and HMOs — a strange and wonderful thing to behold. Here was a nation that had launched, only twenty years prior, a grand new experiment, one in which pharmaceutical companies and its new surrogates in PR and marketing had joined doctoring as an equal partner. Many signs indicated that this new road was a hugely promising one, with chronic diseases arrested and life-spans, or "healthspans," enhanced. The new synergy of marketing and pills — it *had* transformed medicine, and patients! All around the country, people were proactively initiating clinically appropriate prescription switches. Why? Because they could. The nation's newspapers were chock-full of paid and unpaid testimonials to the new age of pharmaceuticals. Yes, there were cynics and carpers and they could make things unpleasant occasionally. But the days when the industry had to worry about "whether there would even *be* an American pharmaceutical industry" — that seemed to be ancient history.

Now the only question was really: What were the limits?

The Full Price

What Living in Pharma's World
Means for Our Bodies

CAN WE TAKE IT? Can our bodies withstand the rise of pharmaceutical power, particularly the kind of power wielded in the new, synergistic way? To restate that "way": using new media freedoms to create chronic disease awareness, using political and regulatory power to speed the approval process, using technology to stimulate demand by stimulating patients and doctors, and then using patient information and marketing to make the patient a partner in a lifelong relationship.

First: How does today's increased, lifetime use of powerful prescription drugs affect the most important human organs? There is no single answer. After all, bodily organs change as one ages. They possess varying levels of tolerance for foreign substances in general (and drugs in particular) and perform differently depending upon one's genes, environment, and behavior. In short, my liver is not your liver — something a drug does not "know" until it's already down your gullet. And therein resides problem number one for any population that plans to use prescription drugs as the first option in treating chronic disease. Why? Because the liver is physiological ground zero for Generation Rx.

It is, for most, a fairly arcane organ; we have a vague idea that it somehow "detoxifies" the blood, but there the folk knowledge usually ends and the discussion shifts to the weather, the wine, the latest vitamin supplement being hawked by Dr. Phil or Dr. Lamm. The liver is not the heart, the emotional centerpiece of modern medicine.

Yet for thousands of years, the liver dominated medicine. To the Hindus, the Chinese, the Greeks, the Romans, the Arabs, and the early Renaissance Europeans, it was considered the main player in determining one's health. Medical thinking in those cultures focused — and in the case of the Chinese and Hindus, still focuses — upon the balancing of bodily humors (bile, phlegm, and the like), which the liver regulates. It was also believed that the liver controlled blood flow. European medicine began to abandon that model in the late Renaissance, when mechanistic notions about how various organs worked began to dominate. Then, in 1628, William Harvey published *De Motu Cordis*, his thesis about the heart and the circulation of the blood. The book slowly sailed Western medicine in a tack toward the heart, a direction that has yet to change significantly. (Harvey's book was described by one eighteenth-century physician as spelling "the end of the sanguine empire" of the liver.) That the heart is allied in fiction and in everyday emotional life with positive things — love, joy, charity — further propelled the organ's ascendancy at the expense of the liver, which lacked a strong, "reason-based" medical lobby. That the liver was often called things like the *porta malorum*, the "doorway of disease," was hardly a recommendation for a promotional T-shirt.

Here is a liver primer: A triangular, three-pound mass of highly specialized cells and ducts, the liver sits in the upper right-hand quadrant of the abdomen, just below the breastbone. It is fed blood via two sources, oxygen-rich blood from the heart via the hepatic artery, and nutrient-rich blood from the gut via the portal vein. The liver does hundreds of things with and to this great stew. The most important include the making of glucose for cell nutrition and the storage of excess sugars as glycogen; the creation of blood-clotting factors, so we don't easily bleed to death; the circulation of bile into the gut to break down nutrients into usable form; the metabolism of proteins and fatty acids; and the processing of all foreign substances into nontoxic waste, which is later excreted into the gut via tiny channels in the liver called bile ducts.

When it comes to drugs (as well as to alcohol or any environmental toxins), this excreting function is the most important. The liver's main cells, called hepatocytes, take drugs, which are fat-soluble, and add another molecule, making them water-soluble, and hence excretable. We can get rid of them. The fate of the hepatocyte is, then, the fate of the body, at least concerning drug-induced problems. As all drugs are, to the liver, a "poison," so all drugs go through this process. But some drugs are more toxic and demanding of the hepatocytes than other drugs. And sometimes the waste product, or metabolite, from drugs is itself deeply toxic, injuring the liver and other organs. Taking drugs in larger quantities, and for longer, continuous periods of time, jacks up the overall lifetime burden on the liver, also known as the "hepatic load."

When the liver becomes distressed, so does the rest of the body. If a drug maims too many cells that are responsible for glucose production, you will suffer from low blood sugar and become fatigued. If the drug clogs up the bile ducts, you will become jaundiced, a sign of severe liver dysfunction. If a drug kills too many hepatocytes, it causes liver scarring, or cirrhosis, which can eventually impede almost all liver functions. If the drug molests the liver cells that process ammonia, a naturally occurring chemical in the human body, a person can become disoriented and, in the case of "fulminant hepatic failure," die. If a drug impairs the liver's ability to make clotting factors, a patient can bleed to death. If the drug kills too many liver cells that process toxins, those toxins can back up into the bloodstream and injure other organs. Death can come swiftly, or slowly.

Yet the liver is also a resilient thing, a true physiological marvel. It is the only organ that can, with time, regenerate itself, a kind of Donald Trump of the human body. Problems ensue when the rate of damage to the liver exceeds its ability to do so, or when other organs have become so thrashed as a result of liver dysfunction that they cannot recover. Then the spleen can bloat from backed-up toxins. The esophagus will bleed backed-up blood from the portal vein. The brain will swell. The belly will bloat. Eye nerves fry.

The challenge is predicting whose liver will be injured by what drug. That is no small task. The liver is in many ways a highly individualized organ — its ability to perform is influenced by things not under our control. This trait is known in medical literature as hepatic idiopathy. Some people have genes that make them better liver-enzyme producers, in turn making them good drug processors. Others have the reverse problem, while still others come with preexisting medical problems that complicate the picture.

But one thing is clear. In the new age of pharma, the liver is under attack, perhaps as no time in modern history, and some of the most respected voices in toxicology and hepatology have stepped forward to sound the alarm. While complete liver failure is still somewhat rare in the United States, liver *injury* is soaring, and drugs comprise an increasing percentage of the assault. As John R. Senior, a veteran FDA expert on the subject, put it recently, "People are taking more and more drugs, both under prescription and by personal choice of OTC remedies, in addition to dietary or nutritional supplements . . . Perhaps as a consequence, drug-induced liver injury has become the leading cause for removal of approved drugs from the market, and for acute liver failure in patients evaluated at liver transplant centers in the United States."

Neil Kaplowitz, the coeditor of the most recent, comprehensive medical textbook, *Drug-Induced Liver Disease,* has even more fun news. "In the United States drug-induced liver disease is the most common cause of acute liver failure . . . a more frequent cause . . . than viral hepatitis and other causes." He goes on: "The frequency and economic impact . . . is a major problem for the pharmaceuticals industry and the regulatory bodies, especially since the toxic potential of some drugs is not evident in . . . clinical testing." Kaplowitz, a professor at the University of Southern California, is particularly worried about the need for better testing, to which there are huge barriers. "To identify acute liver failure [in a new drug] with 95 percent confidence," he writes, "would require 30,000 study patients." Today most new drugs get by, thanks to the reforms of the 1980s and 1990s, with about 3,000.

What has been pharma's reaction? The industry is on the record as opposing any major requirement for expansion of trial populations. After all, they like to point out, about half of drug-induced liver injury, DILI for short, is caused by overdose of over-the-counter acetaminophen (like Tylenol), either intentionally (suicidal) or by "therapeutic misadventure" (among people who mindlessly take a handful a day for chronic pain). But that response is at best a dodge of the facts: an increasing percentage of DILI is provoked by prescription drugs, many of them the very prescription drugs for chronic diseases that we increasingly rely upon as lifelong helpmates and that *we take properly, according to our doctors' instructions.* There are painkillers that cause acute hepatitis, blood pressure meds that block up bile ducts, antidepressants that cause hepatocyte damage, COX-2 drugs that run up liver enzymes and cause artery damage, and diabetes medications that inflame the liver so badly that people die. Some have been removed from the market. Others are on the cusp of such an action. And some are sending up increasingly strong signals that they, too, are making the *porta malorum* very *malorum* indeed.

So, how, specifically, is the liver fairing in Gen-Rx America? How does the business and regulatory system produce and approve a drug that would harm this and other organs so deeply? And who, typically, gets hit? The answer is as close as one's parents' medicine cabinet.

MRS. MORGADO'S LIVER

Every night, Concepción Morgado, a sixty-two-year-old grandmother living in Brooklyn, did something anyone who has ever cared deeply about someone else instinctively understands: she waited up for her spouse to come home from work. Concepción was an admitted worrier, a "very emotional" one at that, but one with a reason for her worry. Several times in the past, her husband, Lazarro Morgado, had been mugged while walking home from his swing-shift job as a janitor; once, it had happened not far down the street from where the couple lived. She remembered how Lazarro had come in the door that night, beaten and frightened. And so, peering down from their third-floor apartment window, Concepción would wait, half sentry, half penitent, sometimes until one-thirty in the morning.

The Morgados had had a long, rewarding marriage. Difficult, true. Fraught with surprises, and not all happy. They had been married in Cuba when Concepción, orphaned at age three and raised by an uncle, was just fifteen. In 1978 the couple immigrated to the United States with their three children because "we did not like the system" in Cuba, she recalled. Life in the United States was better, but not easy. She raised the kids, cooked, cleaned, worked in an apparel shop, took home piecework, and made wedding gowns on the side with her sister-in-law Florinda. As a new *abuela*, she rose to the role, walking her grandchild A.J. to school and back, cooking for the extended family, and making clothes to fill the new financial gaps. Lazarro, a member of Local 32, endured. The work was hard, but it was a job and, strange for the times, it was always there. *Siempre.*

In August 1997, Lazarro said something that only a spouse of many years can get away with saying. "Your breath," he told Concepción one night, "it's really . . . *bad.*" Concepción, a type 2 diabetic, decided that the problem might be the drug she had been taking, Glucophage. On her own, she discontinued it, and then scheduled an appointment to see her longtime physician, Dr. Lara. The halitosis was gone, but Dr. Lara, who had a friendly but frank demeanor, immediately raised an eyebrow when confronted with his patient. Looking at her blood tests, he said: "Your blood sugar is totally uncontrolled." And she knew what that could mean: fainting spells, numbness and infections in the hands and feet, blindness, worse. Yes, yes, she said: She had tried the lifestyle changes in diet and exercise, but the rice and beans — how could one not eat that? "You're going back on the drugs," Dr. Lara told her, and prescribed a light dose of Amaryl. In his notes he also wrote: "Will increase to 4 milligrams, then try Rezulin?"

At the time, Rezulin, Tony Wild and Parke-Davis's sexy new entrant to the diabetes field, was less than nine months into its first year on the market. But sales were already soaring: Rezulin was a poster child for the new, post–Hatch-Waxman pharmaceuticals industry. The drug had benefited from every innovation — legal, medical, regulatory, financial, and marketing — that the era offered. Its review had been expedited via the new, industry-friendly regulations at the FDA — regulations designed to show Congress and pharma that the agency deserved to continue to receive the industry user fees upon which it increasingly relied. The justification for Rezulin's approval had been supported by high-level researchers at the National Institutes of Health, who were, because of the Bayh-Dole reforms of the early 1980s, also allowed to take money from Parke-Davis as consultants on the drug.

Rezulin had benefited from the new, open-door policy at the FDA as well; Parke-Davis executives had extensive contacts with scientists who reviewed the new drug application for Rezulin. The contacts between company and agency were so close that, as court papers would later show, FDA administrators felt totally at ease sending Parke-Davis copies of internal documents in which the chief medical officer reviewing Rezulin said that the drug was no good, that the data was "a pile of shit." That back-channel line of chatter gave the company a way, in other communications, to marginalize the man and his views. Just prior to Rezulin's approval, Parke-Davis also benefited from the industry's new trusting relationship with the agency's scientific advisory committee meetings; according to court documents, company scientists had been able to present their case without filing all of the detailed clinical reports on side effects usually required. It was enough for them to promise to do so later.

And, when it came to marketing, Rezulin emerged as the ultimate pioneer in the new era of pharma synergy. To make sure that the drug was adopted quickly, Parke-Davis's marketing people had used every tactic imaginable to "drill down" to both physician and patient. They floated an extensive thought-leaders program, in which high-writing diabetes prescribers were paid to speak about the drug. There was a faux "research" initiative in which physicians who switched patients to Rezulin were paid for submitting "notes" about each case. There was a Rezulin "preceptorship" program, in which doctors were paid in return for letting a Parke-Davis sales representative tag along on daily rounds. And then there was the patient. In what was hailed as one of the company's more progressive moments, Parke-Davis decided to target Latinos. The company perceived them as an underserved market that was easily influenced. The campaign — "Rezulin: Una Vez al Día" (Rezulin: Once a day) — was soon plastered in and around every barrio bus stop, big-city clinic, and immigrant doctor's office in the nation, including Dr. Lara's.

But Dr. Lara was an exception in one important regard. When it came to prescribing new drugs, he was very old-school. He liked to wait a few years before trying something new. He liked to see more clinical data, more detailed reporting of real-world side effects, and reports of how the drug worked with other drugs. He specifically remembered the Oraflex experience of the early 1980s, when Lilly had heavily promoted a pain drug that turned out to be highly toxic. This he liked to talk about in a colorful, colloquial way. "I mean I had experience with medications like that from since I was a resident, in which they promise you the world and then a lot of patients end up dying. They always like to promise you the world, but . . ." He was not anti-innovation. One of the drugs he had prescribed in the past for Concepción, Glucophage, was relatively new in the United States as well, but there were much better data on its safety and efficacy because it had been in use in Europe for decades. When he wrote, in Concepción's workup, "try Rezulin?" it was the question mark, not just the name of the drug, that mattered to Dr. Lara.

In May 1998, eight months after seeing Dr. Lara, Concepción was not happy. The drug that the doctor had prescribed, Amaryl, made her breath sour, and she began to think that perhaps she should see a diabetes specialist. A number of her friends had been to see a Dr. Salas, a respected endocrinologist who knew and had worked with Dr. Lara. Concepción went to Dr. Salas, who had been heavily detailed by Parke-Davis. Salas had been reassured about Rezulin because it had been approved, only a few months prior, for a new indication: to be used with other drugs, or to be used on its own, as monotherapy. But Dr. Salas did not know — she could not have known, in fact — that said new indication had been obtained with (let's say it, as would a jury, dozens of scientists, and FDA regulators) bogus safety data. A diligent physician with a large number of patients, Dr. Salas would later testify that she would have thought more than twice about Rezulin if she had known the true number of patients in clinical trials who had come down with liver injuries. But when Concepción Morgado's case seemed to indicate Rezulin, all Dr. Salas knew was that it was an effective, popular drug that simply required monthly liver testing in order to ensure its safety. She wrote the script. Concepción filled it and began taking Rezulin.

There were, at first, signs of remarkable progress. Concepción's blood sugar seemed to be better controlled. Liver testing later that spring and summer indicated that she had few elevated enzymes — one of the classic measures of whether a drug is causing liver damage. Both patient and physician were reassured. And why shouldn't they be? That July, Parke-Davis had sent out a "Dear Doctor" letter, discussing liver issues. Although the company knew at the time that liver testing had not warned of liver failure in one clinical patient, who had died, it continued to assert that such tests were valid. There were other troubling signs: the Brits had pulled Rezulin for safety reasons, but, as Tony Wild saw it, that was only because there had been a relatively small market for it in the United Kingdom anyway, making it "easy for them to take the high road in safety matters." In the States, though, Rezulin sales continued to boom. Concepción took her meds diligently.

Then, on August 29, Lazarro arrived home to find Concepción deeply ill. She had been vomiting all day and complained of a pain in her upper-right abdomen, where the liver is located. Concepción was a fairly stoic woman. As Lazarro later put it, he "could tell" if she was in pain, but "she would not say it." Now she was saying it. "When I got up, all the energy flew down," Concepción later recalled. "And I was very yellowish. The whole body: the nails, the feet, the hands." Quickly Lazarro took her to Dr. Lara's — Dr. Salas was out of town — and there learned the shocking diagnosis: she was jaundiced, and her liver cells were dying at a rapid rate. The Rezulin had so damaged her liver that her life was imperiled. She would have to discontinue the medicine and go to the hospital immediately.

The next day, laid up and connected to the frightening ganglia of modern emergency medicine, Concepción's condition slipped. Her state was, medical reports said, "life-threatening." Her liver had nearly stopped functioning. Dr. Salas and Dr. Lara knew that somewhere between 10 and 50 percent of all patients with drug-induced jaundice and elevated liver enzymes die. For ten days, they did everything they could to prevent liver failure. The family gathered around her bed, girding for the worst.

And then her liver panels — the blood tests that indicate how fast liver cells are dying — began to drop. Concepción rallied and spoke of the future. The enzymes fell some more, and more. The jaundice faded. She was discharged and went home. In a few months, her liver panels were normal. On paper, she looked good. Dr. Lara put her back on both of her original diabetes drugs, Amaryl and Glucophage.

In real life, however, Concepción Morgado was a fundamentally changed woman with a fundamentally altered liver, and she would never quite return to the fulfilling, active life she once led. She was plagued with two debilitating conditions: a chronic upper-abdomen pain and endless fatigue. She no longer could walk her grandson to school, or make wedding gowns, or even, many days, cook for Lazarro. As Dr. Lara noted in court testimony, "Number one is the fatigues that she has, intermittent fatigues, the recurrent pains, the loss of outlook in life. I see her personally changed, [from] outgoing and happy and working and enjoying her life and her foods, to somebody that appears that she doesn't know whether she is going to live another day or not. She is very afraid even of taking new medications that might be beneficial to her. So yes, I could say there is a lot of change." His diagnosis: ongoing hepatic insufficiency. Her liver doesn't perform its basic tasks the way it once did.

But the most telling sign of change took place at night, when Lazarro returned from work. "She doesn't wait for me today. She is asleep."

She is also . . . fortunate. By 1999, some twenty-nine people had died from Rezulin-based liver failure, nine required liver transplants, and hundreds more had suffered severe liver injury. Many were in the Latino communities that Parke-Davis had targeted. There were FDA hearings, which resulted in new warnings, but the drug was kept on the market until 2000, when it was recalled because newer, ostensibly safer insulin-sensitizing competitors were approved.

Who was to blame? In the Morgado case, clearly it was Parke-Davis and its parent, Warner-Lambert. That is what a remarkably clear-minded jury found in 2003, when it awarded the Morgados $2 million in damages but refused any punitive award. Warner-Lambert, it found, "intentionally and recklessly misrepresent[ed] or omit[ted] material information about Rezulin to physicians in Dr. Salas's position prior to and during the time Mrs. Morgado took the medication, [and] that misrepresentation or that omission [was] a substantial factor in causing Mrs. Morgado's injury." Worse: "Warner-Lambert act[ed] wantonly and recklessly with regard to Rezulin so as to show conscious indifference and utter disregard for the safety and rights of others." The company had lied, and it had almost killed Mrs. Morgado.

Yet let us also remember two facts: one, that, as Professor Kaplowitz writes, "All the . . . signal[s] were present" when Rezulin was first approved; so why had the system failed? And, two, that Concepción Morgado initiated the switch to Rezulin because her husband told her she had bad breath.

Rezulin was not the only product of the post–Hatch-Waxman era to be pulled or "voluntarily" withdrawn for causing liver problems. Duract, a painkiller made by Wyeth and approved in 1997, is a textbook case of what might be called "too many open doors" at the FDA, and for the wrong kind of drug. There were twenty other analgesics already on the market when Duract was approved, and the senior reviewer at the agency, while he thought the drug worked well at relieving pain, was worried about the fact that many patients in the clinical trials had tested positive for elevated liver enzymes. In a series of meetings with his superiors, the reviewer argued that Duract deserved to have a special "black box" warning about such dangers posted at the top of the label, emphasizing that the drug was safe only if taken for ten days or less. He argued that physicians needed to recognize the gravity of the Duract safety recommendation.

Wyeth, fearing that such a label would severely limit sales, objected. To make its case — and to overwhelm FDA staff arguments — they hired as a team leader none other than Hyman Zimmerman, the world-renowned expert in hepatology and the author of the most-cited medical school text on the subject of drug-induced liver injury. Zimmerman was so respected by the acting director of the FDA division responsible for Duract that, as the *Wall Street Journal* later noted, "He liked to tell people that he still quoted a Zimmerman article written in the year he was born." The results of the Wyeth-FDA meetings, and high-level negotiations with the agency's head of drug evaluation, then under intense political pressure to get approval times down, were somewhat predictable. The ten-day warning appeared, but in tiny type, in the nineteenth paragraph of a fifty-six-paragraph label included with the Duract packaging.

Almost no one read it. Within months, pharmacies were reporting that more than 15 percent of Duract prescriptions were for more than the recommended limit of ten pills. Some prescriptions were for as many as 360 doses, a sign that physicians were prescribing it, in bulk, for chronic pain, for which it specifically was not approved. As sales took off late in 1997, Wyeth detailed physicians heavily. Soon pharmacists were swamped with orders for Duract. Yet when they asked customers if they knew anything about the recommendation that they get their liver enzymes tested regularly, most were clueless. The result was catastrophic. Within a year, there had been four deaths linked to Duract-induced liver failure and eight liver transplants. In June 1998, less than a year after approval, Duract was pulled from the market.

Less than a year — for an agency that was and is severely underfunded, and whose reviewers are under constant pressure to proactively interface with industry, the FDA handled Duract pretty efficiently. In the case of Serzone, an antidepressant approved in 1994 that was flagged early as a severe liver toxin, it took ten years — and eleven U.S. deaths — for withdrawal. No one can quite account for that, given that the drug, which sold upwards of 4.5 million prescriptions a year, was one of the least efficacious antidepressants in that sector's boom market of the 1990s. Even its manufacturer, Bristol-Myers Squibb, claimed that Serzone was mainly for people for whom all of the other antidepressants did not work. Yet its hepatotoxicity was clear, and reports during the years immediately after its release, both at the FDA and at Squibb, indicated that people were suffering from it. Worse, Serzone was a potent liver enzyme inhibitor, which meant that it prevented the liver from processing other drugs properly, leading to further injury from everything from statins to other central nervous system drugs. Yet it was other nations that acted on that information long before the United States did. The Europeans banned Serzone in January 2003, and even the Turks took it off the market before Squibb withdrew the drug in the United States in June 2004.

It would be wrong, of course, to say that neither the FDA nor the industry cares about patient safety. Billions are spent yearly in its service and improvement, and there are thousands of talented, impassioned individuals, many of them driven by professional and social ideals, in search of better patient safety. But it would also be wrong to think that the system as it exists today — lots of industry input combined with stretched agency resources and institutional compromises — is working when it comes to protecting the liver — or any other organ — from bad drugs. That powerful, virulent brew often stifles the ability of the agency to protect the public by institutionalizing lessons it has learned in the past. Instead, the FDA becomes a raft of splintered factions, with the one binding element being the industry's input.

Consider the strange case of Dr. David Graham, a veteran epidemiologist for the FDA's Office of Drug Safety and a noted expert on drug-induced liver injury. Graham is now best known as the FDA renegade who blew the whistle on Vioxx. But his legacy is longer and deeper than that, if only grudgingly acknowledged. It is Graham who is credited with the adverse-event reporting and tough-minded analysis that led to the withdrawal of Rezulin. His methods are now studied by a new generation of drug safety students in universities around the country. Yet Graham, still at the FDA, has found the going rough when it comes to using the methods of that success in reassessing drugs that have already been approved.

One such drug is Arava, or leflunomide, made by Aventis for rheumatoid arthritis and approved in 1998. By 2001 Arava had generated a substantial number of liver injury reports, and European drug agencies were well on their way to restricting its use. The FDA was quiescent until Public Citizen, under Dr. Sidney Wolfe, filed a petition to withdraw the drug, citing eleven deaths from acute liver failure and dozens of hospitalizations. The advisory committee charged with arthritis drugs looked at the rate of Arava-linked liver injury reported in the FDA's adverse-event reporting system (AERS) and found the risk-benefit ratio of the drug to be "acceptable." Graham undertook the same evaluation — and more — and disagreed. Citing the fact that only 1 to 10 percent of severe adverse events are ever reported to the agency in the first place, he performed a complex calculation showing that Arava's rate of injury was likely much higher. Then he got even more aggressive. His division convinced IMS, the giant drug data company that tracks prescription sales, to give it Arava's usage figures for two major health care chains. Graham mined that data to snag a sample of how many real-world users of the drug were reporting liver problems. He then assessed the efficacy of Arava compared to existing drugs. His conclusion, a devastating twenty-two-page memo to his superiors, was that Arava should be withdrawn. "The levels of risk," he says now, "exceed those of Rezulin — and the numbers dwarf Rezulin." About half a million patients a year were going on Arava by 2003.

But Graham was not allowed personally to present his findings to the FDA safety committee on Arava. Instead, his memo was provided with cover letters by the head of the original review committee that approved the drug. Those letters vigorously spun Graham's warning and downplayed its recommendation. "We could not understand why David was not allowed to present," says Public Citizen's Larry Sasich. The committee's "data was straight out of the drug maker's database, which represented people who were being carefully watched and tended to. David's was a view of the real-world harm of the drug, where people are not so carefully tended and treated." Arava was kept on the market, and remains there to this day.

Graham holds a pointed interpretation of the experience. "Everyone [at the Arava safety committee meeting] came from a reviewing background," that is, people who read and approve new drug applications, he says. "I was the only one from a drug-safety background. The reviewing-division background predominates in safety meetings. All these guys have their names on [the drug's approval,] and they are vested in it; they have signed on to its safety and efficacy." There is something else at play as well, he says. Ever since PDUFA was passed, an increasing number of NDA reviewers have been put on year-to-year contracts. "They get subjected to an incredible amount of pressure to change their opinions," he says. "I'd like to know what percentage who say no to a new drug are renewed."

There is one way that an individual's hepatic reaction to a drug can be predicted, or at least approximated. That method involves the scrutiny of a key, drug-metabolizing enzyme system in the liver known as cytochrome P450. (Pay attention: this is not as hard as it sounds, I swear.) For the last decade, CP450 and its numerous subsystems have become the intense focus of academic pharmacologists because science has been able to identify the main genetic traits that lead to varying degrees of CP450 sensitivity. Some genes lead to increased sensitivity to some drugs; some genes lead to decreased sensitivity. The next logical step is to take these insights from the lab and expand them from generalizations about various populations (for example, Latinos' CP450 genes make them bad metabolizers of alcohol) to more specific tests for individual and group susceptibility to liver poisoning. And to do that, a growing cadre of scientists say, drug companies should invest heavily in drug-gene identification.

The promise of such an investment is rich, according to Alastair Wood, the editor of the *New England Journal of Medicine*'s influential drug reviews section and one of the preeminent drug safety experts in the world. Wood is no antipharma rabble-rouser. As he sees it, drug-gene identification would benefit the industry and the patient. "Dosing [the determination of how much of a drug can be optimally and safely administered] is the single most important decision in creating a good clinical trial because you will be locked into it later [on the label]," he says. "By doing early genotyping you can identify responders versus nonresponders" — people with varying degrees of drug-processing abilities. And that would not only make the drug safer for the patient, but also could expand the use of some previously thought to be overly toxic substances. "I think that drug companies should get out of the pills business and just do this," he says.

Yet he has found little response to his ideas from mainstream pharma. Genetics is an expensive, lengthy road for any company to take, as evidenced by Jan Leschly's folly at SmithKline a decade ago. Moreover, it does not fit into the quarterly stock report mentality that dominates the pharma investor community. But Wood believes there is another source of resistance. "The drug companies are scared to death of it because it makes risk more predictable on the label," he says. And the more precise you are about risk on the label, "the more difficult it is to market."

It pays to note that Wood is hardly being esoteric in his concerns. Several other drugs — many wildly popular — have substantial hepatotoxity, but their merits have been judged to outweigh such deficits. COX-2 inhibitors (Celebrex, still on the post-Vioxx market) and statins (among them Lipitor and Zocor) are two of the biggest-selling classes of chronic disease drugs, and liver testing is recommended for both; they are nowhere near as toxic as Rezulin, but they will need to be scrutinized ever more intensely if they are to remain controllable. Both are the

subject of enormous scientific and marketing campaigns to expand the percentage of Americans who take them. Hence, the
liver remains on the front line.

THE HEART, THE LUNGS, THE GUT

Yet the liver, for all its centrality, might best be seen as the ca-
nary in the mineshaft of Generation Rx. In terms of outright
numbers, other parts of the human body — the heart, the lungs,
the gut, and the brain — routinely suffer the most severe adverse
effects of the new era's new ways with pills, and none of these organs is as resilient as the liver.

The heart in particular gets whacked: A fist-sized organ made
up almost entirely of muscle, the heart is remarkable by any
fathom of the imagination. It pumps blood through the body sev-
enty-plus times a minute, twenty-four hours a day, for (if you are
lucky) a long, long time. To understand its miracle and vulnerability, think of the heart as a pump. The heart has a motor —
thick muscles that contract, or pump — that is fired by an energy
source, a cluster of cells called sinoatrial nodes, a kind of natural
pacemaker. If a drug interferes with the firing of these nodes, say,
by blocking the flow of key enzymes and minerals, the pump can
become erratic, as if it had no surge protector. The pump has external plumbing — arteries and veins — that move the blood in
and out, and an internal system of its own to keep it nourished.
Drugs that block those pipes, or thicken their inner lining, can
cause a backup and a blowout; drugs that interfere with the
pipes' natural equilibrium processes — the arteries' way of keeping small internal bumps from rupturing and blocking the pipe
— can do the same. Such events are called heart attacks, among
other things. The heart pump has valves that open and close with
pistonlike regularity; they are part of the motor, in a sense, as
they help guide blood to the right place and prevent it from
backflowing to the wrong place. But if a drug compound with tis-
sue-toughening properties interferes too often, the pump strains,
puts a heavier load on other heart and lung functions, and can
even shut down from overwork.

The diet drug Redux was a grim case in point. Marketed by American Home Products (AHP), Redux worked by stimulating the release of the neurotransmitter serotonin, leading to appetite suppression. Unfortunately, Redux stimulated too much serotonin, and in the wrong organs — in the heart and in the lungs. That excess serotonin provoked two harmful events: first, it caused a thickening of heart valve tissue, and second, it evoked a similar thickening of the blood vessels that run through the lungs and into the heart. It made the pump strain and break down. The result: within a year of Redux's release, patients were dying from a form of high blood pressure known as primary pulmonary hypertension.

And again, the problem was not just that the drug itself caused injury, but that Redux was, just like Rezulin, very much a product of the new way of getting prescription drugs to market and quick profitability. As with Rezulin, the process, instigated to help both shareholders and patients, became a vehicle of harm for both. Redux's approval was speeded by FDA staffers who had direct connections to American Home. Justification for its approval was based on the popularization of the real consequences of unchecked obesity, but that premise also served to obfuscate the drug's substantial lack of efficacy and to gloss over safety issues. Its approval was speeded, too, by pressure to improve FDA review times by Congress and the industry, which held a gun to the agency's head through PDUFA fees. And Redux was, like Rezulin, a phenomenon of the mass media, both paid and free. It was the subject of a huge, $52 million advertising campaign. (The company's public relations firm even created a mascot for the drug, Roxanne Redux, to establish its brand image quickly.) Redux became a billion-dollar blockbuster in its first year on the market.

The increasingly familiar nightmare followed, courtesy of the new synergy. When safety concerns about Redux arose, American Home's medical consultants wrote positive reviews for the drug and got them published in prominent medical journals without fully revealing their financial ties to the company. When the FDA advisory committees took up the safety concerns, they were lobbied heavily by industry and its Washington, D.C., power brokers. When FDA staff scientists told AHP what they really thought of the drug's safety profile, they were sidelined, and lectured by their superiors in the agency about being "too blunt."

Today, the consequences of Redux are still being felt by patients and their families. Some 45,000 patients have reported either heart valve damage or primary pulmonary hypertension, both of which are debilitating and often fatal conditions. For American Home, the consequences were dire as well. The company was almost put out of business because of billions in legal settlements on Redux claims.

Yet Redux was hardly alone in the ranks of drugs suspected of causing heart damage. As studies showed that more than 10 percent of all adverse drug reactions reported to the FDA were cardiovascular in nature, several drugs were either voluntarily withdrawn or ordered off the market. Then, in 2004, Vioxx, Merck's vaunted COX-2 painkiller, along with Pfizer's COX-2 drugs, became the biggest nonwar and nonelection story of the year.

Recall the original promise and intent of the so-called coxibs: Unlike other anti-inflammatories, COX-2s were approved by the FDA and justified by their makers based on the notion that they were easier on the gut. For a small portion of people taking traditional anti-inflammatories for arthritis pain — aspirin, naproxen, ibuprofen — that was important; these patients indeed had gastric bleeding, gastric congestion, and ulcers, which were antagonized by the older nonsteroidal anti-inflammatory drugs, or NSAIDs. Clinical trials showed that such patients might be better served by the COX-2s.

But the initial COX-2 promotional campaigns went much further. It was suggested, repeatedly both in the media and in ad campaigns, that the new drugs were also better at controlling pain. They were "superaspirins." The skating star Dorothy Hamill was drafted for a new campaign promoting Vioxx for osteoarthritis. "This is my favorite time to skate," Ms. Hamill said in a commercial. "I guess it's from all those years of five A.M. practices. But it's also the time when the pain and stiffness of osteoarthritis can be at their worst." The result was that a new, expensive drug once intended for a fairly small population became the expensive default prescription for most forms of adult arthritis pain, while many less expensive and equally effective drugs fell by the wayside. By 2002, 74 percent of people taking COX-2s were *not* considered to be at risk for ulcers. They had received these prescriptions simply because the drugs were new. Even pro-industry research groups concluded that heavy promotion was behind excessive prescribing of coxibs.

The hype — and the "superaspirin" prescribing binge that followed — served to steamroll important safety concerns about the drugs' impact on the heart. This phenomenon applied especially to Vioxx, the brand name for Merck's rofecoxib. Vioxx was the symbol of Ray Gilmartin's new, improved, superfast Merck. (Recall that the company often bragged that "in the United States, just four days after FDA approval, the new medication was already being shipped to customers. Eleven days after approval, more than 30,000 pharmacies had shelves stocked with Vioxx.") Yet, early on, independent researchers worried about it. In 1999, one prominent team showed that an unintended effect was that COX-2s disturbed the ability of the arteries to prevent little internal bumps from exploding and turning into a blockage. Others noted that coxibs like Vioxx (as well as Pfizer's Celebrex and Bextra) posed something of a therapeutic dilemma. By selectively inhibiting only the COX-2 enzyme, they were able to alleviate pain without causing gastric problems (the COX-1 enzyme is responsible for gastro-protection). But as it turned out, COX-1 was also responsible for raised levels of blood clotting — it was *good* to inhibit it, especially if you were older or inclined to heart problems. Increased blood clotting was often the cause of heart attacks. That was why people taking the older painkillers — from aspirin to ibuprofen — had lower rates of heart attack and stroke. Merck knew that by giving up aspirin and taking Vioxx, patients could be putting themselves at increased risk of heart attacks. The company's solution? Patients with cardiovascular risk profiles who were taking Vioxx should also take a daily low-dose aspirin.

In 2001, the FDA castigated Merck for that recommendation. Taking aspirin with Vioxx canceled out the gastro-protection that was the *sole reason* for taking Vioxx over aspirin in the first place. Worse, the age group most likely to take Vioxx was also the age group with the highest cardiovascular mortality. "The potential advantage of decreasing the risk of [gastrointestinal problems] was paralleled by the increased risk of developing cardiovascular . . . events." The agency then went on to warn Merck not to use promotional materials that minimized the risk of heart attacks from Vioxx use.

Merck complied, but its backbone, now that Vioxx was the company's biggest revenue generator, stiffened. It was going to fight other sniping at the drug with legal guns if necessary. That resolve went on broad display in 2002, when the company sued a Spanish pharmacologist for criticizing the drug. Writing in the Spanish-language pharmaceutical journal *Bulletin Groc,* Juan Ramon Laporte, of the Autonomous University of Barcelona, published a critique of COX-2s entitled "The Alleged Benefits of Celecoxib and Rofecoxib: A Scientific Fraud." Laporte's most damning point — and it was based on the work of one of Europe's most eminent and independent clinical-trial scholars — was that Merck had minimized cardiovascular events in the clinical trial it had used to win FDA approval, a trial known as Vioxx Gastrointestinal Outcomes Research, or VIGOR. Merck's response was to sue Laporte and the journal's publisher, insisting that they be ordered to run a correction for false allegations against Vioxx. In 2004, after two years of consideration, the Spanish court found for Laporte and the *Bulletin*, dismissing Merck's claim and ordering the company to pay the defendants' costs. The International Society of Drug Bulletins issued its own statement, saying that the journal article "accurately reflects the reports of serious methodological deficiencies and irregularities" that surrounded VIGOR and Vioxx.

The evidence against Vioxx piled up. A study of nearly 380,000 patients in Tennessee's Medicaid program found, for example, that users of Vioxx were about 1.7 times more likely than nonusers to have congestive heart disease; among new users of the drug, the rate went up to 1.93 — almost a doubled risk. That was one real-world representation of what was going on with Vioxx. By August 2004 researchers in *The Lancet* were reporting even more dire results. Vioxx "was associated with an unanticipated fivefold increase in myocardial infarctions compared with naproxen. Further, more recent studies with rofecoxib have shown its propensity to raise blood pressure and its capacity to precipitate CHF [congestive heart failure]." And that wasn't because the patients weren't taking their aspirin. It was because of something specific to Vioxx, perhaps related to the way it affected blood fats and made them stickier.

After evaluating the pros and cons of the drug, *The Lancet*'s editors then issued a stunning manifesto against Vioxx, a summary of which took up the entire cover of the journal. It is worth quoting at length: "The coxib field had been marked by intensive DTC advertising in the United States, and sales of these drugs exceed $7 billion a year. Yet it is hard to imagine the justification for this extraordinary adoption of coxibs in light of marginal efficacy, heightened risk, and excessive cost compared with traditional NSAIDs . . . The continued commercial availability, without a black box warning for [heart disease] patients, is indeed troubling."

Troubling, yes. And for the hearts of the elderly, even more so. But Merck was silent. It was not until two months later, after it released its own study, that the company would act. The study had been concluded and its results known a year earlier: it showed a doubled risk of heart attack in a population of Vioxx users who were also at risk for colorectal polyps. The company later justified its suppression of these findings by saying that the results were preliminary and limited to case studies, not an actual clinical trial. Thus Vioxx remained on the market until October 2004, one more daily drug in the national apothecary of harm. By then, it may have caused upwards of 140,000 cases of heart disease and between 56,000 and 100,000 deaths. Pfizer's Bextra, one of its COX-2 inhibitors, remained on the market for another six months, until the FDA ordered its removal in April 2005. Pfizer's other coxib, Celebrex, remains on the market despite deeply troubling signs that it too is a harmful drug.

What about the two classes of drugs specifically created by the industry to extend the life and health of the heart? How have they fared — and how have we fared under them?

If there is a major success in the new pharma realm so far, it is the statin, the cholesterol-reducing agent that first emerged from the laboratories of Merck in the 1980s. Statins work by inhibiting something called coenzyme A, which helps the liver build cholesterol. Cholesterol is an integral part of the greater cell-tissue building process, but too much of it causes the arteries to clog. Slowly but surely, large epidemiologic studies have proven statins' worth in slowing that process by cutting cholesterol production and reducing inflammation. Three such reports have shown that statins, when taken on a daily basis, decrease the risk of second heart attacks by 30 percent and the risk of death from second heart attacks by 40 percent. Perhaps just as important, in a society geared toward reducing risk, are so-called primary prevention studies involving statins. These have shown dramatic drops in the development of cardiovascular disease in people with high cholesterol but no history of heart problems. In other words, statins can prevent heart attacks in seemingly healthy people. And direct-to-consumer ads appear to help — albeit expensively — at getting more of those people (and their physicians) to adopt the drug. Bob Ehrlich's notion of making the campaign for Lipitor "all about the numbers" might not have been such a bad idea after all. About 10 million Americans now take one of five approved statins.

But that success has come with its price as well. In 2000, the statin known as Baycol, made by Bayer, was removed from the market for causing thirty-one deaths from rhabdomyolysis. All statins carry some risk of "rhabdo," a sudden and devastating weakness of the muscle tissue; as it turns out, the same statin action that inhibits coenzyme A also suppresses other vital cell-maintenance enzymes, particularly one that maintains muscle and heart tissue. So far, the rate of true rhabdo has remained very low. About one in one thousand patients will experience some form of the disease, which almost always remits when the statin in question is discontinued. Baycol, unfortunately for those who took it, provoked a severe form. More recently, a new statin,

Crestor, has come under attack by the same researchers and public health advocates who blew the whistle on Baycol for causing
a similar reaction while providing no better results than existing,
proven statins. AstraZeneca, the maker of Crestor, has chosen to
fight such charges, investing millions in a public relations and ad
campaign to establish Crestor as the next blockbuster statin. It is
too soon to tell what will happen.

There is also the concern that wholesale adoption of statins essentially causes people to indulge in imprudent lifestyles — a
kind of "I'm on Lipitor so give me my Big Mac and shut up" mentality. It is not hard to find anecdotal examples of this reality, but
there is little money to be found to carry out research that goes
beyond the anecdotal, and one wonders about the consequences
of a conclusive study that showed that the very option of a statin
somehow induced people to party on.

The most reasonable worry when it comes to statins is what
will happen if vast new numbers of patients begin to take them
in higher doses. It is almost inevitable that such will occur, as
both the government and industry have been pouring billions
into research on the effects of cholesterol reduction and heart
disease prevention. In 2004, one foreshadowing of that effort
made front-page news. The NIH, backed by the top heart-related
medical organizations, dramatically revised its recommendations for desirable cholesterol levels in those at moderate and
high risk for heart disease. Citing five large studies, the researchers said that statin therapy for those at moderate risk for heart
disease should commence when their low-density lipoprotein
(LDL), or "bad" cholesterol, exceeds 100 on any given lab test.
The previous cutoff was 130. That meant that millions of Americans not previously considered candidates for statin therapy
would now be hearing from their physicians that they should begin to take the drugs. Just as important, and perhaps as troubling,
is the aggressive dosing the new recommendations suggest. In
the past, physicians would start a new patient on a low dose of
statins and settle for small improvements in blood fat tests. The
new recommendations advocate drastic reductions — 30 to 40
percent — and hence administration of larger doses.

(A not-so-small note: Eight of the nine experts on the NIH panel recommending expanded statin use had received financing from one or more statin maker.)

Yet it is at higher doses of statins that problems are more likely. A recent study of Zocor, Merck's statin, showed that aggressive, high-dosage treatment produced only moderate changes in cholesterol. But the change in dose, from forty milligrams to eighty, more than quadrupled the risk of developing rhabdo, from one in a thousand to a more troubling four in a thousand. Four people in every thousand adds up, especially if you are constantly adding new millions to the ranks of should-be statin takers. (Lipitor, Pfizer's statin, did not register such risks at the higher dose.) And for a class of drugs that require daily, lifetime usage, there are surprisingly few studies of long-term use. All of which shows that the statin, the new era's poster boy for heart health, is very much a work in progress. And there lies a chief irony of the new pharma age: to be the nation at the edge of new discoveries, we must be willing to be part of the experiment.

The other great inventions of late-twentieth-century pharmocapitalism were drugs for hypertension, or high blood pressure. High blood pressure — which can cause everything from heart attack to stroke — is a leading cause of premature death, and its causes are complex, ranging from too much salt to obesity. In essence, hypertension puts undue pressure on the heart, lungs, and other organs; using the pump analogy, hypertension would be akin to putting a lakeful of water into a pump designed only to handle a small pond. The number of Americans said to be afflicted with hypertension ranges into the tens of millions; the number of untreated does as well.

Recall now the promise of ACE inhibitors and calcium channel blockers, which make blood vessels open wider, leading to reduced pressure. They would be so free of side effects that patients would be more compliant, and so would have their hypertension better controlled — a key to better heart health.

Unfortunately, such drugs — and the promotional campaigns that drove their ascendancy — are slowly emerging as some of the more problematic of the new era. Not only did they drive up the cost of treating hypertension, but they may well have caused more harm than good. Consider a five-year study, issued in 2002, of more than 42,000 patients. In it the National Heart, Lung, and Blood Institute (NHLB) did something the industry had long refused to do. It compared the use of diuretics — the older, cheaper, unpatented medications for hypertension, which worked by reducing water retention — with the newer ones, like Pfizer's Norvasc, a calcium channel blocker, and Merck's Prinivil, an ACE inhibitor. What it found was remarkable. What the nation had got back for billions in increased prices for the new drugs was — worse results.

The ACE inhibitors fared most poorly. Compared to participants who took diuretics (at $25 a year), those who took the new drugs (at $250 a year) registered two points higher on the top end of the blood pressure reading, with African Americans indicating four points higher. How did that play out in terms of real-life medical consequence? Compared to the water pill takers, the ACE takers had a 15 percent higher risk of stroke overall, with blacks at a 40 percent higher risk. Furthermore, the risk for heart failure was 19 percent higher, with the risk of requiring surgery 10 percent higher among ACE takers. Those taking calcium channel blockers (at $500 a year) fared little better. And the unnecessary economic costs were staggering. In one review of prescription patterns, diuretic use declined from 56 percent in 1982 to 27 percent in 1992. If diuretics had been allowed to maintain their market share, the study noted, the health care system would have saved $3.1 billion.

How had that happened? Nearly every major researcher in the NHLB study chalked it up to one thing: the enormous amount of money spent on marketing the new drugs, money in the form of ads, and, perhaps more importantly, money spent on studies that trumpeted the new drugs without comparing them directly to the older ones. Here the pervasiveness of pharma money was stunning. In a *New England Journal of Medicine* review of seventy medical journal articles on calcium channel drugs, 96 percent of authors in favor of the drugs had financial ties to pharma. Of those who were critical of the drugs, only 37 percent had such relationships. All of which suggests that, when it comes to the human heart, the new synergy was not always heart-friendly.

The lungs are a frail organ, yet they are the port of life itself, as it is through the lungs that we take in the oxygen that fuels and re-vivifies our blood supply, via a complex system of airways, called the bronchi. They terminate in little sacs, which come into contact with blood vessels and pass on fresh air, oxygen, and pass out spent air, or carbon dioxide.

It is also through the lung's blood vessels that we metabolize many of today's most advanced pharmaceuticals. One consequence is a startling rise in the numbers of drugs with the potential to cause pulmonary disease, a number that has risen from 19 in 1972 to 150 in 2002. Many are predictably toxic, such as drugs for acute conditions — cancer treatments, for example. But many are drugs for chronic conditions, from heart drugs to drugs for pain, and they are not so predictable. Most of their toxicity is provoked by what lung specialists call a "hypersensitivity reaction." It can be caused by a wide variety of factors, from genetic predisposition to preexisting conditions. The usual symptoms include difficulty breathing, cough, and fever. Sometimes there is tightness in the chest.

Somewhere between 3 and 20 percent of all patients taking ACE inhibitors develop a hard, dry cough, requiring termination of the drug for complete recovery. Enzymes that ACE drugs inhibit for the purpose of reducing blood pressure are the same enzymes responsible for reducing spasms of the bronchi, the main air-supply network of the lungs. When the bronchi spasm, you can't breathe. Other drugs can be even more lung-toxic. Amiodarone, a drug used to treat heart arrhythmia, has been shown to cause severe lung diseases, from interstitial pneumonitis — swelling of the spaces between the lung's air sacs, causing oxygen starvation — to solitary lung mass. Methotrexate, a common drug for treatment of rheumatoid arthritis, can weaken the lungs' natural protective pathways and allow for opportunistic infections. Aspirin and traditional anti-inflammatories can also encourage bronchial irritation by inhibiting COX-1, which, as it turns out, is also responsible for slowing down bronchial stress. Some nasal sprays, particularly those known as alpha-adrenergics, cause interstitial fibrosis and obliteration of pulmonary vessels, which is as bad as it sounds. And Relenza, the anti-flu treatment that Glaxo's Bob Ingram so agilely fought the FDA over, turns out to cause serious bronchial problems in people with asthma and other respiratory disorders, especially in the elderly and in children.

There are also drugs — many widely prescribed, some not so — that are serious suspects for pulmonary toxicity. The most intriguing and troubling of these are the SSRIs, which, because of their passing resemblance to Redux, the diet drug whose serotonin-releasing properties caused primary pulmonary hypertension, have fallen under recent scrutiny. There are, to be fair, very few cases of SSRI-induced fatalities from pulmonary failure. But there is a persistent pattern, and it has not, so far, received much attention from the health media.

The same can be said for a number of other drugs: there is no money for seemingly obscure drug-safety issues. But there are risks. In January 2004, the Japanese Ministry of Health announced that there had been five deaths of drug-induced interstitial pneumonia in the four months since Arava, the controversial drug for rheumatoid arthritis, was launched there. The drug was considered an apparent cause in two of the deaths and was being investigated in the other three. Worldwide, there have now been eighty cases of Arava-associated pneumonia.

The stomach is a courageous organ, both for what it does (breaks down nutrients in preparation for processing by the rest of the intestinal tract and then the liver) and for what it puts up with in the process (fast food, the stress of modern work culture, and gas, gas, gas!). As such, the modern gut is the martyr of the contemporary corpus, Saint Gastronomica with arrows. It is hardly surprising, then, that this same organ suffers from increasing use of pharmaceuticals.

One of the great innovations of the new pharma era was gastrointestinal medication, H2 blockers and proton pump inhibitors.

These ulcer drugs are the kind that Glaxo's Ernest Mario so cleverly "repositioned" to treat something called GERD, which used to be called heartburn. Such drugs — from over-the-counter Tagamet to expensive prescription drugs like Nexium — have become huge sellers, the mother's milk of pharma annual reports. They, perhaps more than any single category of pill, help keep the stock price of a pharmaceutical company in the double digits, and the stock itself in our retirement portfolios. They are one of the purest confections of the synergy era: recall that GERD drugs do not reduce GERD by correcting its true cause — that the esophageal sphincter loosens and allows stomach acid into the esophagus, thereby creating the burning sensation. Rather, they "cure" heartburn by suppressing stomach acid. The industry sold this fix by focusing on the notion that the real problem was "too much stomach acid," which is not the case. The drugs have been accepted by the public for obvious reasons: they allow us to indulge in fatty, sugary foods without paying the price, and they allow us to lead stressful, work-focused lives with less discomfort. As the drugs themselves are harmless, traditional critics of the industry have paid them little attention.

Yet a small but growing body of literature is calling the use of GERD drugs into question, particularly the daily, long-term use indulged in by about 2 percent of Americans. That translates to about 2.5 million daily long-term users. The question for their guts is: What are the consequences of chronic suppression of stomach acid? After all, acid and alkaline — in balance — are absolutely crucial to the proper functioning of the stomach. The stomach is designed to maintain that balance, both to provide a neutral site for digestive enzymes to do their work on food and as a barrier to foreign bacteria, which can cause all kinds of metabolic havoc and disease.

Among the most concerned about GERD drugs is Dr. Jonathan V. Wright, a clinician at the Tahoma Clinic in Kent, Washington. For almost three decades, Wright has been treating patients with a variety of chronic diseases, and for years he has tracked something strange and troubling: Many people who presented with digestive problems were also chronic users of GERD drugs. They had been told that too much stomach acid was bad and had come to rely on the drugs to keep the heartburn demon away.

Yet, as Wright knew, too *little* stomach acid can be just as bad as too much; in fact, it can be worse. It can, for one, lead to a severe lack of properly digested minerals — minerals essential to the health of all key organs. Often he saw the consequences to patients in late middle age — folks who would come in the door dragging, listless, and wondering why they were feeling like Ozzy Osbourne looks. (Sorry, Ozster!) A simple blood test that Wright performed usually explained the symptoms: the patients were dangerously low in B_{12}, folic acid, calcium, and zinc. Their rates of anemia were high, too — a sign that they were not getting enough iron to allow their blood to transport oxygen. Worse were the lowered amounts of folic acid and B_{12}: they provoked higher levels of homocysteine, an amino acid implicated in heart disease. The low zinc levels were causing premature eye degeneration. It was not pretty.

Following his nose and medical training over prevailing wisdom, Wright undertook two main courses with such patients. First, he took them off *all* GERD drugs. Second, he put them on regimens of mineral supplements and hydrochloric acid, which would bring up the level of acid in their stomach. In almost all cases, the patients' problems resolved themselves. "It was revealing in so many ways," Wrights says. "The prevailing wisdom had accumulated so much to the point of view of the manufacturers that we have forgotten the basic fact: that stomach acid is good for you."

Are Wright's success and insights purely localized, the result of one impassioned, dedicated physician who focuses like a laser, or do others in the medical establishment share such views? The answer can be found in recent work on a phenomenon called bacterial overgrowth, which happens in the stomach when the pH balance — the balance of alkalinity and acidity — is continuously out of whack. One of the stomach's jobs is to act as a sort of barrier to germs coming in from above (in the form of things like salmonella) and from germs coming from the intestines below. When there is not enough stomach acid, the stomach itself is transformed from a relatively neutral environment to one in which germs grow. The consequences are twofold: we become more susceptible to infection, and the germs steal nutrients and make it difficult for us to properly metabolize fats, vitamin B_{12}, and carbohydrates. At least nine studies, from 1996 through 2002, show that chronic use of acid-suppressing drugs results in bacterial overgrowth, with several implicating the condition in common diseases of the elderly.

Even more hair-raising is preliminary work that suggests a link between GERD drugs and the development of a condition known as atrophic gastritis, in which the stomach can no longer secrete enough acid to protect itself from infection. In a study published in the *New England Journal of Medicine* in 1996, researchers from Sweden and the Netherlands wrote about how they had followed two groups of patients who were being treated for reflux. One group took Prilosec, which suppressed acid production; the other underwent surgical repair of the esophageal sphincter, which does not cause acid suppression. Many in both groups also had *Heliobacter pylori* — the bacteria that cause ulcers. The results were eye-opening. Of the Prilosec patients who had *H. pylori*, the rate of atrophic gastritis went from 59 percent to 81 percent. Of those undergoing surgery, the rate was 4 percent.

No one knows exactly how atrophic gastritis causes stomach cancer. It may be because it results in the circulation of too much gastrin, a hormone with strong links to the development of such cancer, or it may be because of the way in which acid suppression promotes bacterial overgrowth and an environment ripe for chronic inflammation and infection. One thing is clear: acid suppressors are increasingly viewed with suspicion by those concerned with stomach cancer rates. As Dr. Julie Parsonnet of the Stanford Medical School wrote of the Swedish-Dutch results, "In principal, current [acid-suppressing drug] therapies might be advancing the cancer clock by converting relatively benign gastric inflammation into a more destructive, premalignant process." To be sure, she added, there was, as yet, no convincing evidence that acid-suppressing drugs raise the risk of gastric cancer, but "the long-term use of acid-inhibiting therapies in patients with *H. pylori* infection should be viewed with some caution."

Dr. Wright believes much more work needs to be done on the cancer connection, but he is convinced that Generation Rx will increasingly pay a high price for its current use of GERD drugs. "People will end up with diseases in their sixties and not associ- ate them with the consequences of long-term acid suppression," he says. "It is a slow, insidious thing, and we do not pay attention to it."

In October 2004, two of the nation's leading gastroenterolo- gists issued an unprecedented warning: people who chronically use GERD drugs should be aware that they are more vulnerable to pneumonia-type infections.

YOUNG BODY, OLD BODY

Again, can we take it?

And who, specifically, suffers the most from pharmaceutical harm — harm that might be averted if the present system were changed? What if clinical-trial results were reported fully, or new drugs were not pushed with such force? Or regulators were sim- ply left to regulate instead of being "proactive partners" with pharma on what are often only marginally safe and effective, me- too drugs? The most common victims are the young and the aged, and, of course, the parents and children who take care of them. Today, their stories are legion, and they are increasingly moving off the easily dismissed "victim" and trial-lawyer Web sites and onto the front pages of the nation's most esteemed newspapers.

First, a primer about young and old bodies: in a word, they are changing. The young are still developing key organs, muscles, and bones; the elderly are experiencing organ deterioration. In both cases, these organs — from the brain to the liver — metabo- lize and dispose of drugs in less than predictable ways. But be- cause clinical trials do not tend to focus on such populations, steering a demographic middle course for both marketing and scientific reasons, little is known about how many drugs will affect the young and the old. As an article in *Pediatrics* points out, "More than 70 percent of all *Physicians' Desk Reference* entries have either no existing dosing information for pediatric patients or explicit statements that the safety and efficacy in children have not been determined."

No one group has discovered the darker aspect of this information void as have the parents of children and adolescents taking antidepressants. One of them is Mark Miller. In 1997, Miller, a middle-aged advertising executive, and his wife, Cheryl, moved into a new suburban neighborhood outside Kansas City, Missouri. It was a big move, even if they were just switching suburbs. Their children, Matt, thirteen, and Jenny, fifteen, had to change schools, and for Matt, a slender, usually easygoing boy with fine features and an all-American tousle of blond hair, that was anything but easy. During the first year at his new middle school, he grew withdrawn, and his teachers, suspecting something more than early teen blues, suggested that the Millers seek professional help, which they did. As Mark Miller recalls, "We were advised with great authority that Matt was suffering from a chemical imbalance that could be helped by a new, wonderful medication called Zoloft. It was safe, effective, only two minor side effects were cautioned with us — insomnia and indigestion." The physician, who, unbeknownst to the Millers, had served as one of Pfizer's "thought leaders," gave Matt a week's supply of the drug and told Mark and Cheryl to call "when you know how Matt is doing."

Almost immediately, Matt's demeanor seemed to warp. He grew easily agitated and could not sit still. He would not eat, and he wasn't sleeping well either. But the doctor had warned about the sleeplessness and possible stomach upset. And the ups and downs of their teenager, no matter how unlike himself he seemed, the Millers tried to take in stride. After all, Matt still seemed to be interested in all the things that usually engaged him; he had a new video game, and he was looking forward to the family vacation, which was to commence that coming Monday.

But such was not to be. The night before the family was to depart, after taking his last Zoloft tablet, Matt Miller killed himself. His father found him. As he tells it, "Matt hung himself from a bedroom closet hook, barely higher than he was tall. To commit this unthinkable act, something he had never attempted before, never threatened to any family member, never talked about, he was actually able to pull his legs up off the floor and hold himself that way until he lost consciousness and forced himself to leave us." Matt's autopsy showed the levels of Zoloft in his blood were three times the therapeutic minimum levels, despite the standard dosage he had taken.

The Millers, devastated for years, slowly looked for the answers to the inevitable questions: How could such a thing happen? Why? Are we alone? They began to network on the Web, where, upon contacting other parents, they began to find the answers, or at least some of the answers.

Certainly they were not alone. There were scores of parents with similar stories. Common in all of them was the intense violence of the suicide or suicide attempt, the fact that the youths had not been on the antidepressant very long, and that no one had warned them that SSRIs could cause a condition known in the medical literature as akathisia, a state of internal restlessness and agitation so intense that taking one's life can appear to be the only way to relieve it. Often, parents had been counseled to "be persistent" in the face of a child's initial trouble with the drug. More often than not, the prescriber was a general practitioner with no training in psychopharmacology.

Such was the case of Jake Steinberg, a twenty-year-old college senior and accomplished pianist. Steinberg had gone to an internist to get a referral to a bone specialist for sore hands. As his mother, Alice, recalled, "The internist who saw him for thirty minutes prescribed Paxil because he bit his fingernails, and the doctor thought it might help with that." Like Matt Miller, Jake Steinberg began to behave erratically. He stopped sleeping. His stomach ached. Then, a few weeks later, while at work at an internship he had earned in New York, Steinberg began exhibiting bizarre behavior. One day, he ran through the offices, threw a chair through a window, and then, in a final, concerted act of despair and agitation, threw himself to his death twenty-four stories below.

There were other tragedies. There was twelve-year-old Caitlin

McIntosh, an A student who killed herself eight weeks after being started on Paxil and then switched to Zoloft; she hung herself by her shoelaces in the girls' bathroom of her middle school. There was seventeen-year-old Julie Woodward, who hung herself in the garage of her home seven days after the start of her Zoloft regimen. She had no history of self-harm or attempted suicide. And there was young Cecily Bostock, a recent college grad who, two weeks after beginning to take Paxil, got up in the middle of the night and, using a large chef's knife, fatally stabbed herself, twice, in the chest. Her mother, Sara, recalled: "This was a young woman who had everything to live for. She had just completed applications to grad school and received a large pay increase the month before. She had a boyfriend who loved her and scores of wonderful friends. She had never been suicidal."

Then there was Justin Cheslek, twenty, who went to his college health service complaining of insomnia. After a workup, in which the physician noted "no suicidal ideation," Cheslek received a prescription for Paxil. When he complained that he didn't like the way it made him feel, he was put on Effexor. Within twenty-four hours, he had a seizure. Five days later, he hung himself in his apartment. As his father recounted the details to an FDA advisory committee: "He didn't leave a note. Beneath him were his laptop computer and a glass of Coke. It was as if some sudden impulse had made him do this. We grilled his girlfriend about his mood and behavior in the months prior to his death. She said his demeanor changed dramatically around her birthday, February 22. Justin started taking Paxil February 21."

Akathisia was not the only unrevealed side effect at play in many of the suicides and suicide attempts. Withdrawal syndrome — a sudden, intense, flu-like syndrome often accompanied by both mania and depression — also loomed large in both young and older SSRI users. But parents had not been warned about that either. At SmithKline, Paxil had been relabeled eleven times before there was any mention of withdrawal, and then only in a deeply buried paragraph. The company's chief, Jan Leschly, himself once brushed aside a question about the process by saying that "some people will never get enough information."

But how had SSRI use become so common among children and adolescents in the first place? None of them were FDA-approved for such a purpose, and the few studies that had been done on pediatric depression and SSRIs were equivocal at best on their effectiveness in younger populations. The answer might be summed up the way a movie might be pitched: Pharma's new synergies had merged with the modern health care system. DTC and off-label had met HMO and managed care. Start with the fact that depression among all populations is a real medical issue. It has become easier to diagnose, and seeking treatment does not carry the stigma it once did. Add to that the fact that managed care makes more traditional talk therapy unavailable to most people; recall that HMOs like Kaiser routinely indicate that drug therapy is the first-line course of action for most diagnosed cases of depression. (It also happens to be about one fourth as expensive as talk therapy.) Multiply this imperative by the entire panoply of modern pharma marketing, from the paying of thought leaders to influence peers to try meds for unapproved uses, to outright off-label marketing, to the museum exhibits that authoritatively proclaim that depression is caused by a chemical imbalance, to the "depression awareness days" routinely underwritten at high schools by all the major SSRI makers. And remember: Paxil was initially targeted as a half-billion-dollar-a-year drug. It was Jan Leschly's "stretch goals" that made it a mass-market blockbuster, a pharmaceutical Twinkie.

Yet that *is* the system, one we seem stuck with, and certainly one that few seem ready to alter substantially. So the real issue to the SSRI parents was: Why didn't anyone tell us about these potential side effects? And it is here that even those who continue to believe in the usefulness of antidepressants overwhelmingly fault the industry. The most charitable read it as a case of fragmented decision making and regulatory numbness. Others assert that it was all about maintaining sales. Whatever you believe about motivation, you can be certain that every major SSRI maker fudged when it came to reporting publicly the rate of suicide, suicidal ideation, and violence associated with use of their drug. Such was the conclusion of David Healy, a professor of medicine at the University of Toronto and the only independent researcher to look at every single SSRI study ever done. Speaking to an FDA advisory panel convened in 2004 to decide whether to place a prominent suicide risk warning on antidepressants, Healy, who still believes in the therapeutic value of well-monitored SSRIs, delivered a damning set of data. "There have been 677 trials involving SSRIs," he said, "and having helped review all of these, I can let you know that roughly only a quarter of the suicidal acts that have happened in these trials have been reported in the scientific articles that have come out of those trials."

There were all kinds of duplicity and institutional leniency at work as well. Healy recalled that when SmithKline originally submitted Paxil suicide figures to the agency in 1989, they indicated an eight times greater risk of suicide for adults on Paxil than for those on a placebo. But the FDA, already getting an earful about suicide risk and Prozac, was worried about the "public relations" effect of such figures, and wrote SmithKline, telling the company to resubmit its data. As a number of court cases now reveal, SmithKline reran the numbers, giving the drug a more benign profile. Paxil sailed to approval. As Healy noted, "They were only doing what Lilly and Pfizer had already done."

Mark Miller and David Healy's advocacy, and that of hundreds like them, eventually made a difference for future generations of children and parents confronted with possible antidepressant use. In October 2004, the FDA ruled that it would require all makers of antidepressants to underscore the risk of suicide by placing a black-box warning on each and every prescription. No one referred to it as a victory.

Yet one question — still largely unanswered — has continued to swirl around the subject of children and adolescents vis-à-vis psychiatric drugs. Why do they seem to display vulnerabilities not displayed by adults? Why does their akathisia play out as suicide and not, say, as generalized anxiety disorder? Many believe that a clue lies in the stimulating nature of most antidepressants, and in the evolving brain structures of the young. About 90 percent of a person's hard wiring develops before he or she reaches the age of twenty. The process is known as myelination — the coating or insulation of nerve networks that protects them from crisscrossed signals from other neurons. Childhood and adolescent brains are thus highly plastic. Any foreign substance that interacts with such malleable cerebral structures — in the case of SSRIs, for example, the brain stem — might impede or diminish their functioning, causing them to act unpredictably. (One of the few imaging studies of adult Paxil users, for example, showed that it causes important changes in the brain-stem region.) Changing brain structures might thus magnify the stimulant effect of such drugs. That stimulant effect might be the unanticipated, frightening burst of energy that allows someone who is merely thinking of suicide to take sudden, dedicated, and violent action. Instead of cutting oneself, one hangs oneself — an act long recognized as one of the most serious, intentional acts of self-harm. In self-hanging, one is willing to hurt — hurt deeply and for a considerable length of time — before one dies.

Brain plasticity looms as a concern in the long-term use of any psychiatric drug. It is, however, an area of great neglect. The industry does not sponsor studies of long-term use, even though it supports and popularizes the practice of lifelong dosing. (When it does underwrite pediatric studies, about 25 percent show that either the dose must be changed to prevent adverse events noted among children, or that the drug did not work at all.) No one really knows just what that will mean for a new generation, who will be relying not just on SSRI drugs, but also on Ritalin and its imitators. The frontal lobes of the brain, which manage feeling and thought, do not mature until age thirty. Will prescription drug use alter those key structures? Speaking in a recent *Time* cover story, the noted University of California, San Francisco, expert on child psychopharmacology Dr. Glen Elliott uttered a rare discordant note. "The problem," he said, "is that our usage has outstripped our knowledge base. Let's face it, we're experimenting on these kids without tracking the results."

You might call one rising element of that trend "pharmaceutical creep" — the growing off-label use of ever more powerful drugs on children and adolescents who do not respond to SSRIs and Ritalin. The most worrisome is the use of antipsychotic medications to treat children with severe disruptive behaviors. Such drugs, known as atypical antipsychotics because they do not manifest the severe side effects of older versions, have come into vogue because they sometimes work when other drugs have failed. But they are already causing problems, including the development of breasts in young boys, and insulin resistance, the precursor to diabetes, in teens. Another concern: researchers are already experimenting with the prophylactic use of such drugs in children who are the sons and daughters of schizophrenics. These are kids who are totally without symptoms but who have a high risk of developing the disease. A laudable goal it may be, but if it works, the practice — again, using powerful psychiatric compounds on still developing children — will take a lot of monitoring, and one wonders when the health care system will begin to pay for that.

In the realm of clinical trials, children and adolescents have become pure gold, both for the industry and for contract research organizations — including the skunky "health communicators" that "help" people stay in such experiments. There have been more than two hundred pediatric trials since 1998, the year after Congress passed legislation that granted patent extensions for firms that conducted such testing. That, in itself, might not have been a bad idea; tax breaks and patent incentives have their place as goads to innovation. (Whether that place includes the wastebasket has yet to be determined.) But the process is deeply flawed. For some reason, never clearly explained, the new law allowed these pediatric trials to go forward without the same demanding informed consent and monitoring requirements in place for traditional new drug applications. The result was a bonanza for pharma. Between 1997, when the law was passed, and 2001, the number of children in trials increased from 16,000 to 45,000, with the industry spending in excess of $1 billion a year on them. Unfortunately, much, if not most, of this new spending was not for pediatric trials of cancer drugs, but for pediatric trials of chronic disease medications.

Many pediatric trials are run responsibly, but many are not.

Consider the case of Propulsid, yet another pill for esophageal reflux, approved for adults in 1993. Having been heavily detailed about the effectiveness and safety of Propulsid by its manufacturer, Janssen Pharmaceuticals, physicians did what enterprising physicians do: they started trying it for off-label illnesses. Pediatricians, for example, began prescribing it for infants who had chronic acid reflux. Yet Propulsid came with a risk, even for adults. At the time of its approval it was known to cause fatal heart arrhythmias in a small subpopulation. By 1997, when the Pediatric Act was passed, it was already implicated in the deaths of three young children. The FDA insisted that Janssen either test the drug on youth or include a warning on the label. The company pasted on the new warning label and passed on the study. Here is where the story gets interesting: Instead of taking up its own study, Janssen began offering the drug for free to researchers who were doing their studies on childhood gastritis. It is hard to get around one interpretation of that move: Janssen wanted to research-surf, on the cheap.

By 1999, that tack had turned deadly. In November of that year, Gretchen Stevens took her nine-month-old infant, Gage, to a specialist at Children's Hospital of Pittsburgh. Gage had been suffering from chronic acid reflux, which irritated his esophagus and made him cry. It was a condition that he would likely have grown out of by his first year or so, but Gage's specialist recommended that Gretchen place her son in a study she was running for a new drug. That drug was Propulsid. Not long after, Gage died from cardiac arrhythmia. It was caused, according to the official coroner's finding, by the drug.

What other investigators found in the wake of Gage's death was appalling, though in a strange way rather comforting to Janssen. In assessing the cause of the infant's demise, FDA investigators heaped almost all the blame on Gage's doctor, saying that she had failed to report one serious incident involving Propulsid and another baby. "They told me they were just trying to see how effective it was," Gretchen Stevens told Alice Dembner of the *Boston Globe*. "Had I known it was a dangerous drug, I would never have let him take it. Who in their right

mind would?" There was one other damning FDA finding in the
Stevens case: a pathology report submitted just before Gage en-
tered the study found no evidence of "significant inflammation."
Gage did not need the drug in the first place.

By 2000, when it was finally taken off the market, Propulsid
had been linked to one hundred deaths, including those of nineteen children.

Still, one might argue that the Stevens case is hardly the right
exhibit in any brief against pharma's role in pediatric testing.
The trial was not officially sponsored by the drug's manufacturer, the FDA said oversight had been lax, and the place where it
had been performed was a children's hospital in a large urban setting, the kind often stretched for adequate staff and money to do
the job right.

No one could say that about Eli Lilly's clinical trials for Cymbalta, or duloxetine, its successor to Prozac. For years, Lilly had
been testing it in some of the most secure, well-funded research
centers in the world. By 2003, Lilly was so assured of the drug's
impending approval that it hired a powerful New York public relations firm just to walk the aisles of the annual convention of
the American Psychiatric Association and hand out the results
of the studies. The company employed a troop of PR specialists
to work the financial and health press, confidently predicting
that approval was (their words to me) "just around the corner."
Lilly analysts pegged their sales forecasts for Cymbalta at $2 bil-
lion a year.

The hype notwithstanding, by late 2003 Lilly had run into a
number of unanticipated setbacks. One was particularly oner-
ous. The FDA requested that it conduct a new study of the drug
in healthy volunteers — people without depression. Healthy-
volunteer studies are used to determine how the human body
metabolizes a drug and to flesh out proper dosages and side-effect
profiles. The company promptly began aggressively advertising
for volunteers, offering $150 a day for what would likely be a
thirty-day study. The trials would be held at Lilly's own, hotel-
like complex at the Indiana University Medical Center. It was
state-of-the-art in every sense.

Tracy Johnson, a nineteen-year-old student at nearby Indiana

Bible College, was intrigued with Lilly's ads, and in December 2003 she decided to drop out of school in order to partake of the lucrative offer. She needed the money, and the study seemed to provide relative comfort: housing and meals as well as what would be, to any student, a tidy sum of cash. Lilly told her about the risks involved in taking Cymbalta. There had been four suicides over several years of testing, but those, the company stressed, had occurred among patients who were depressed. Tracy was not. Lilly believed that there was no evidence that it might induce suicidal thoughts, a strange assumption given the problematic history of antidepressants, and the fact that, at the time, the FDA had ramped up its investigation of just that issue. Tracy Johnson signed up.

For the next month, she dutifully took her daily dose of Cymbalta. She was cheerful, as usual. She submitted to the blood tests and other monitoring provided by Lilly at its Indiana University research center, where she was free to come and go as she pleased. Over twenty days, her dosages were increased, eventually to five times the recommended dose, and then decreased. Her mood stayed the same. At the end of the month — by then she would have made roughly $4,500 — she was placed on a placebo. Four days later, she spoke with one of her best friends and "sounded happy."

The next evening, she was found dead. A nurse discovered her body in a bathroom of the Lilly complex. She had hung herself by tying a scarf to a shower rod. She did not leave a note.

Why? In the aftermath, a number of suggestions arose. A serious one concerned withdrawal syndrome. Perhaps Johnson, only nineteen, had been a particularly slow metabolizer of drugs in general. That might trigger reactions during the placebo period, later than expected. Cymbalta, after all, is similar to Effexor, which was known for causing severe withdrawal reaction upon discontinuance, and patients experiencing severe SSRI withdrawal had been known to commit suicide. On top of that, Cymbalta had been shown, a year before, to be a potent inhibitor of cytochrome P450, the liver enzyme responsible for processing drugs.

When the Indiana University review board looked into the

case immediately after Johnson died, it did not rule on causality, but, rather, ordered Lilly to discontinue the recruiting operation and, tellingly, to bring in an "independent psychiatrist" to evaluate the remaining participants (nineteen of whom dropped out right after the suicide). The company was also ordered to have patients sign a new consent form. (No one knows what was in it.) Lilly responded with its own investigation, which concluded that the drug was not implicated in the suicide. The Indianapolis coroner ruled the drug out as a suspect, but then later admitted that it had not tested Johnson's blood for traces of Cymbalta. In August 2004, the FDA agreed with Lilly. It approved Cymbalta for treatment of depression, inaugurating one of the biggest new drug launches in history.

I asked Steve Paul, Lilly's chief research and development officer, if the aggressive way in which drugs are marketed now might make patients in trials like Cymbalta's think that the risks were not as high as they truly were. This suggestion Paul brushed aside, but then added, without any prompting: "I think you are saying, 'Should we be careful not to over-incent people?' And you are right. We should not. And we are careful not to."

Children, adolescents, teens, young adults . . . what of the unborn? Such is yet another concern, small but growing, in the vast universe of chronic disease drugs. It is referred to as teratogenic load — the effect of drugs on pregnant women and their newborns. It is not a topic that gets a lot of press. In some ways the United States has been lucky when it comes to prescription drugs and birth defects, escaping the thalidomide disaster of the late 1950s, which was almost entirely confined to Europe. But that was when Europe was faster than we were in approving new drugs. Yet today, even despite faster approvals, the United States has remained relatively fortunate. Chemical assaying and animal testing keep most major teratogens out of the drug supply. (A notable exception is isotretinoin, or Accutane, for acne, which remains on the market, mainly for youth, because there are no other options for treatment of severe acne.) But there is a long streak of luck at play as well.

Will this pharmacological roll of the dice founder? As the sheer volume of drug approvals skyrockets, and as manufacturers get better and better at pushing physicians to adopt new meds faster, experts in the field of toxicology have begun to worry about the limits of their ability to assess risk. Animal studies, the main method of determining teratogenicity, are hardly infallible. There is already a small but surprising group of data concerning statins and birth defects. Physicians are clearly warned on the label of every major statin that pregnant women, and women planning pregnancy, should not take the drug. But statin use has become so widespread, and physician monitoring time has been so dissipated, that keeping an eye on female patients who fit that profile is almost impossible. In 2004, researchers from the NIH performed an intricate data-mining experiment using the FDA database. They found thirty-one cases of rare limb and central nervous system defects in infants exposed to the most popular statins. The researchers concluded that the number of such abnormalities was far in excess of what was expected.

The greater concern, however, is that we are not investing in the systems to adequately monitor teratogens in the drug supply. As Dr. Allen A. Mitchell of Boston's Slone Epidemiology Center writes: "The unfortunate reality is that we learn about virtually all teratogenic effects only after a drug has received marketing approval, and of course, only after it has been used by pregnant women . . . Though a number of individual research programs have been established to generate and test selected hypotheses . . . these programs have not had the mission or the resources for the systematic and routine study of the risks and safety either of drugs newly introduced to the market or those commonly used in pregnancy." He concludes: "Operating without overarching guidance, direction, or support, these programs do not act as a coherent system to ensure the early and effective detection of birth defects caused by drugs in current use."

And so, in the new era of lifelong pharmaceutical use for chronic disease, the youngest and most vulnerable fly without a parachute.

In the supersenior world of Lilly CEO Sidney Taurel, prescription drugs not only ease the familiar pains and complications of aging, but actually extend lifespan and enhance its quality. (Recall Taurel's proclamation about the company's new compounds for osteoporosis: "We are building new bone!") There is some evidence — and it is trumpeted mightily and at great length in a variety of paid and unpaid media — that Taurel and pharma are onto something here. But the reality of prescription drugs and aging, at least when it comes to chronic diseases, is both a little more mundane and a lot more worrisome. Let us consider the real supersenior . . .

Begin with a little trip to the internist with good old dad, for some routine tests, shall we? He's feeling a little achier than usual around the hips lately, and he's been bending your mother's ear about it forever, and you've just taken your Provigil anyway so you're good to go. Vroom, you're off.

In the doctor's office, you're given a medical history form:

"Yeah, we have to fill one of these out again. OK, what meds are you taking?"

"None."

"You sure? Hmm. OK. And when was the last time you were here?"

"I think it was the week before your mother's birthday."

"So that makes it, let's see, November 29 . . ."

"Except for the kidney pills —"

"The kidney pills? But I thought you said you didn't —"

"Maybe it was your sister's birthday, come to think of it."

"Forget that. They have that on your records anyway. What's this thing about a kidney pill?"

"Yeah. The kidney doctor. He gave me some pills after I had my operation."

"When you had your kidney removed, right?"

"Yeah, but there was just one bottle of them."

"And you stopped taking them when?"

"When what?"

"The kidney pills."

"From who?"

"The kidney doctor!"

"I thought this was just a checkup with the regular doctor —"

"It is! I'm just asking about what pills you're taking."

"Oh, I told you. None."

So goes the typical day with a typical aging parent in a typical visit to the typical doctor's office.

Let us now add to this complicated picture something equally complicated but not so charming: the typical supersenior body. It is, to state the obvious, a grand machine that has begun to wear down. In aging, all of the processes that normally handle the metabolism of drugs slow and become more labored. The absorption of drugs is affected, for example, by decreased movement of the intestines brought on naturally by the aging process. (New studies document how chronic use of GERD drugs further diminishes the gut's ability to absorb drugs in general — the very "slow, insidious thing" that Dr. Wright worried about in the 1990s.) Aging also profoundly affects pharmacokinetics, the way drugs move through the human body. Older adults almost always have reduced lean body mass and body water, and increased fat mass. Drugs that dissolve in fat — like antidepressants — thus have a greater half-life; they hang around longer, and so increase the duration of their action. (This is why Valium, for example, should almost never be prescribed to the aged; the buildup of the drug exerts a pronounced effect on cognition, which is why so many seniors on Valium end up confused, debilitated, and frightened.) The decline in muscle mass and water also inhibits the distribution of water-soluble drugs like ACE inhibitors, leading to sometimes dangerously high concentrations. The process known as pharmacologic "clearance," or excretion, slows as well. As the liver and kidneys harden, scarify, and shrink from the natural rigors and excesses of life, metabolism of drugs becomes harder, less efficient, prolonged. That means more time for the drug to cause mischief in any number of organs. All of this is medically complicated, in terms of diagnosis, by one overarching reality: different bodies age at different rates. One man's kidney might be like a thirty-year-old's, his liver that of an eighty-year-old's.

Now add to this natural process the unnatural: the increasing prevalence of polypharmacy — the use of five or more drugs at the same time — among the aged. Here the numbers are truly staggering. In 2000, the American Society of Clinical Pharmacology and Therapeutics pegged the percentage of elderly patients receiving *nine or more* medications at 27 percent, compared to 17 percent in 1997. The figure continues to mushroom. Polypharmacy, to be fair, is not in and of itself a bad thing; as humans age, they are likely to have more than one medical problem, and drugs often can be helpful. But polypharmacy requires more physician monitoring, not less. And less, as anyone who has studied trends in medical supervision knows, is exactly what most seniors (and everyone else, for that matter) will likely get in the world of managed care.

True, it might be argued that physician behavior and managed care policy are not the responsibility of drug companies, but that the content of polypharmacy is fundamentally pharma's charge, and in that regard most drug companies have been about as responsible as a thirsty sailor in port after a year at sea. Most drugs have simply not been tested for use with other drugs. As Steven Werder wrote recently in *Current Psychiatry*, "Most individuals who are prescribed five or more drugs are taking unique combinations, [representing] an uncontrolled experiment with effects that cannot be predicted in the literature."

The uncontrolled experiment hardly seems strange to today's aged and their kin, but only recently has it earned its own name and, hence, official attention — the "prescribing cascade," or simply "the cascade." As the geriatric pharmacologist Lori A. Daiello forthrightly described the cascade in a recent issue of *Psychiatric News*, "A medication — drug number 1 — causes an adverse effect that is interpreted as a new medical condition. Drug number 2 is then prescribed to treat this 'new' condition. Drug number 2 causes an adverse drug effect or interaction, interpreted as a new condition, so drug number 3 is prescribed, and so on." And so on indeed. By 2002, some 28 percent of all hospital admissions of the elderly were due to medication problems, at a whopping cost of $20 billion annually. The cascade is expensive in more ways than one.

In 1999, a professor of geriatric psychiatry at the Medical University of South Carolina named Jacobo Mintzer, along with Alistair Burns at University Hospital of South Manchester in England, began to write about one particularly troubling aspect of the cascade. Could the way seniors were being given prescription drugs actually be a force behind the rising rates of cognitive decline in the elderly? In other words, do prescription drugs, and the way we use them, cause mental impairment, thereby provoking even more unnecessary prescribing? Mintzer and Burns looked at drugs that inhibited acetylcholine, a neurotransmitter that we need for proper brain function. Among such drugs are antidiarrheals, antipsychotics, and older antidepressants, as well as digoxin (a heart drug), codeine (for pain), captopril (another common heart drug), and even high-dose Tagamet (for heartburn/GERD). Of the twenty-five medications most regularly prescribed to geriatric patients in the United States, Mintzer concluded, thirteen have "significant anticholinergic activity at the doses commonly prescribed," meaning that they impede the necessary work of acetylcholine. There is widespread and largely unmonitored use of these meds.

The effects of such drugs are often both devastating and unrecognized in origin. Take cimetidine, a.k.a. Tagamet. Mintzer found that common high doses of Tagamet in the elderly were associated with "reversible confusional states — confusion, delirium, slurred speech, hallucinations, and coma." Worse, he found, many of the principal chronic conditions of aging — angina, congestive heart failure, constipation, diabetes mellitus, urinary dysfunction, sleep disturbance, and dementia — are worsened by drugs with anticholinergic activity.

Part of the reason is aging itself: as humans get older, cholinergic transmission often declines, as does drug metabolism. But just as often the drugs themselves are the culprits. Why is that? Again, the problem is a lack of reliable information. In theory, Mintzer said, a physician should be able to predict the "anticholinergic load" and risks of any combination of drugs. "In practice," he concluded, "the information available from the product label and from published work focuses on side effects of drugs used as monotherapy," or alone. In this deficit, manufacturers were deeply implicated. The long-term consequence of the trend, Mintzer concluded, was nothing short of a "cholinergic bomb."

Lack of information, when it comes to geriatric prescribing, is hardly a new concern. As early as 1991, a group of researchers headed by Mark H. Beers, then at the UCLA Center for Health Sciences, decided to use all of the tools at their disposal — national expert surveys, pharmacy data, and clinical notes — to come up with a definitive list of inappropriate geriatric drugs. As Beers saw it, the list — and the thirty criteria he and his colleagues used to determine it — could then be utilized by internists for review of individual patient regimens. In September 1991, he published the list, then about twenty-eight drugs long, in the *Archives of Internal Medicine.* "The Beers List" was promptly declared the gold standard.

And it was promptly ignored. All through the 1990s, even as the Beers List grew in length, and in esteem, the number of elderly patients receiving Beers List drugs grew. In a 2004 study of 765,000 patients, researchers found that 21 percent of elderly patients had filled prescriptions for drugs that "are known to cause harm or induce harmful side effects in those over 65 years of age." Even more dramatic was the increase in drug-drug interactions and the elderly. An ambitious study of the phenomenon, appearing in the *Journal of the American Medical Association,* showed that 5 percent of all hospital admissions for the elderly were due to drugs "known to cause drug-drug interactions. Many of these could have been avoided." Again, it was all about drugs with *known* adverse effects. The cost: about $16,000 per hospitalization.

What was behind the rising rates of polypharmaceutical injury in supersenior America? And just what kind of reactions are we talking about? Over and over, the experts blamed "inadequate monitoring" by the "system." Such was the conclusion of one study that showed that, despite clear and sustained warnings to the contrary, "More than 40 percent of all benzodiazepines are prescribed to people over sixty-five." In more than one third of all cases, pharmacy computers had failed to recognize and properly warn. There was more: most physicians were — and are — not formally trained in polypharmacy; in the great tradition of all doctoring, from Hippocrates to Osler to Dr. Koop, they learn as they go. But how do they learn? There are few continuing medical courses on polypharmacy for chronic disease management, and most are sponsored by pharma, hardly the objective source most patients might expect. Beers himself was hired by Merck to edit their manual of geriatrics. He remains there to this day, an esteemed pioneer whose thoughtful warnings still struggle to penetrate the walls of modern health care. Beers's message is more crucial now than ever, because polypharmacy *is* complicated, and it is not going away.

Again, what could be driving the polypharmacy injury trend? "Perhaps because most physicians in practice today had little or no training in geriatric medicine, they may simply not be aware of the advances in this rapidly growing field," writes Knight Steel, a professor of geriatrics at the New Jersey Medical School. Or, he asks, "Is there too great a willingness to prescribe drugs on the part of the physician and too great an expectation on the part of the patient to receive them during an office visit?"

Unasked in Steel's rumination is this question: What fuels physician willingness, and what implants great expectations in the first place? What creates pharmaceutical appetite and what might be called the Great Pharmaceutical Default in modern chronic disease medicine? The answer is complex, and I hope I have suggested elements of it more than once so far. But just in case, let me state it as a mathematical equation: if we assign to X the natural inclinations of human beings to avoid suffering and, whenever possible, to take the easy way out; to pp the polypharmaceutical ignorance of many physicians; to mc the parsimony of managed care; and to bs the power of the industry synergy and advertising, we can state the creation of Pharmaceutical Default (PD), thus:

$$X^2 (pp\, mc)\, (bs) = PD$$

Or restate it this way: The problem of the aged and drugs for chronic disease is one of specific physical vulnerabilities meeting a fragmented health care system driven by the marketing imperatives of drug companies.

And so for the aging and the elderly prescription drugs become — often with no geriatric testing at all — a proxy for real medical care, with sometimes devastating consequences. It is a situation almost identical to that of the young.

4

The End of the Great Buffer?

Why We Are More Vulnerable

SO, WE *CAN'T* TAKE IT — at least not without some help. But what kind of help? Our doctors and our government have traditionally served as the great buffer between pharma's excesses and our bodies, and so a tour through those worlds might help us assess how well they can really continue to do that.

SHOES ON FIRE

To understand the doctor dynamic, let us first put ourselves in the shoes of the modern doctor. First and foremost, those shoes are on fire. Managed care, a force for bringing the overall rate of health care costs down, lit the flame, and the extent of the heat now staggers. Today the average physician must see from four to five patients an hour, and there are no signs that those visits will get longer any time soon. Rather, in the near future Kaiser, the California-based managed care pioneer that often sets the pace in such trends, will likely constrict the visits even further. So will its less progressive brethren, who face growing numbers of patients in general, shrinking revenues from federal and state budgets, rising expectations from corporate policy holders, and unrelenting shareholder pressure to do more with less to ensure better profitability. Now add to this intense pressure from within the pressure from without: an aging population with a growing sense of medical entitlement; a younger immigrant population with severe economic and communications problems;

huge spikes in malpractice insurance and a seemingly endless swarm of malpractice attorneys, ready to pounce. Being a doctor isn't so sexy anymore.

Now enter the pharma factor. In 2005, Dr. Average stands as the object of the most intense, seductive, and potentially lucrative marketing campaign in modern history, a $12 billion a year bacchanal that spends between $8,000 and $15,000 annually per physician to sell its wares. The industry's messengers have morphed as well. Gone are the old, fuddy-duddy medical affairs people, the semiretired pharmacists and nurses who spoke so tentatively of new advances. Today the average physician routinely sees pharma reps so young that they still listen to Britney, their youthful ways conjuring, like, more of a pharmaceutical lap dance than, like, an old-fashioned sales call. (A recently published account by a former Viagra salesman, *Hard Sell*, details how female reps allow male doctors to give them back rubs.) There are now 80,000 to 90,000 reps, about one for every five physicians.

More are coming. One of the most popular on-line courses from the Learning Annex is entitled "Three Days to a Pharmaceutical Sales Job Interview!" In the workbook for the course, a former pharma sales representative named Lisa Lane, presents the work diary of Corey Nahman, also a sales rep. Although obviously sanitized for mass consumption, it gives a peep into what doctors encounter daily:

7:45 A.M.   Attend grand rounds at the hospital early in the morning to meet my customers for coffee and a bagel and some friendly lobbying. I might work the room, making pseudo-appointments for later in the day.

10 A.M.   Visit the hospital outpatient clinic to increase demand for my products with the residents and other house staff.

10:30 A.M.   Call on a couple of pharmacies and see how well my products are selling and see if any new doctors have moved into town.

11 A.M.   Call on a local HMO and "twist some arms" in a polite manner, of course.

| 1 P.M. | Take a client out to lunch or bring in lunch for a group of doctors. |
| 1–5:30 P.M. | Call on some of the doctors I saw at the hospital at their private offices. |

When it comes to drugs for chronic diseases, the reps' underlying, unspoken message is equally simple and seductive: this drug will keep patients away from the office.

By almost any measure, Dr. Average has succumbed to that message. That is not to say that he or she is, *ipso facto*, practicing bad medicine, but today one is safe in assuming that there is an unseen presence in the doctor's office. The indicators are unrelenting: One's physician may well be a paid pharmaceutical thought leader, getting $10,000 a pop for speeches to his fellows in which he or she talks up a new medication. She may be getting paid for "case studies" — in essence a copy of your experience (your name extracted) after you try the new drug. And then there are the endless small gifts and grants, the free travel to such medical research meccas as Palm Beach and Jamaica, or to some Mardi Gras–timed "consensus conference" in New Orleans. Being a doctor *can* be sexy again!

The Demi Moore in this lap dance is CME — continuing medical education. CME class credits are required for physicians if they want to stay in good professional standing, but such courses can be expensive. That is why some 90 percent of all CME classes (totaling $900 million in 2003) are currently paid for by pharma. The relationship between CME providers and pharma is, not to put too fine a point on it, close. It isn't all tainted; much is done responsibly and objectively. But it is an exercise in denial to think that CME does not translate into new prescribing patterns, and that sometimes these patterns result in harm, especially for Mr. Liver, Frau Heart, and Señor Kidney. Think Vioxx, Redux, Paxil, and Rezulin.

For the most part, physicians believe that they are immune to these new forces, that their advanced education, advanced social status, and professional ethos serve as a sort of inoculation against bullshit and hype. (The late Dr. Louis Lasagna, a clinical-trial pioneer, revered by both industry and industry critics, once noted that physicians always feel that they are in the "authoritative," or superior, position, until it comes to payment, "when suddenly they see the patient as an equal.") But a growing body of literature, addressing what Massachusetts General's David Blumenthal has dubbed "the gift relationship," points to an opposite conclusion. Even small gifts, the endless pens and notebooks, for example, impose a sense of indebtedness on physicians. One study looked at whether the value of the gift mattered. It did not: "Feelings of obligation," the authors wrote, "are not related to the size of any initial gift or favor." Although this concept might run counter to what the never-ending spate of penis-enlargement ads on the Internet suggests, it makes perfect sense when you think about it. As Blumenthal says, humans "have trouble seeing themselves as biased when the bias serves their needs or advances their own perceived interests . . . To posit otherwise would imply that physicians are different in fundamental ways from their fellow human beings."

The biggest indicator that pharma is sitting next to the patient on the examination table is the industry itself and how it spends its cash. Simply put, industry money out nets even more money in. Detailing works. Consider off-label prescribing, which has skyrocketed since the court rulings that established pharma's right to distribute off-label data — studies, say, paid for by GlaxoSmithKline to show how great Paxil is for twelve-year-olds. "Incentivization" of physicians also works. That is what marketing executives at Schering-Plough discovered not long ago, when they simply began mailing out unsolicited $10,000 checks to leading liver specialists. The checks were consulting fees that required nothing other than that the physician agree to prescribe Intron A, Schering's drug for hepatitis C. The physicians were also offered $1,500 a head for each patient put on Intron A and entered into a clinical trial for the drug. The trials required little more than the writing up of case notes; patients and their insurers, however, had to pay for the costly drug. Sales went through the roof. Intron A, it should be noted, is far from a state-of-the-art drug, and its efficacy in treating hep C is still sketchy. Its adverse effects, like that of most hep C treatments, are severe.

All of this connotes unseemliness at best and neglect of duty at its worst. But is anyone really hurt? Certainly the answer is yes if you recall young Matt Miller (Zoloft) and Caitlin McIntosh (Paxil, Zoloft), grandmother Concepción Morgado (Rezulin), and the infant Gage Stevens (Propulsid). The same goes for off-label prescribing of chronic disease meds in general. Today the FDA says that at least 8,000 people a year become seriously ill because of it. Since physicians report only about one in ten such instances to the agency, the figure is in reality more like 80,000.

Less dramatic but far more extensive is the harm to the tradition of patient-physician independence. In a review of sixteen studies of drug company–physician interactions, Dr. A. Wazana found that "the resulting changes in the use of medication were often costly and nonrational in that the newly prescribed or requested drugs had no therapeutic advantage over the alternatives." Repeat: Costly and nonrational. Wazana then went on: "Interestingly . . . the larger the number of gifts that physicians received, the more likely they were to believe that gifts did not affect their prescribing behavior." As a social scientist might say, gifts create arrogance. Physician attitudes, pharmaceutical entrepreneurship, and managed care now conjure a new golem, the invisible, patched-together "other" of the modern examination room.

OUT OF SIGHT

In addition to doctors, the other great buffering force is government — the FDA, which regulates new drugs; Congress, which funds the FDA and holds subpoena power for all pharma records; and the White House, which appoints the officials who are supposed to oversee the process. Together they constitute what now passes for the nation's pharmaceutical prophylaxis. They are all institutions fundamentally mediated by politics, some more so than others, and in the last ten years they have all had their old buffering powers blunted by pharmaceutical company political activity.

No one has been more integral to the industry's political success than Alan Holmer, the head of PhRMA from 1996 to 2004. Like Gerry Mossinghoff before him, Holmer is a classic Reaganite, one best known for his role in negotiating the U.S.-Canada Free Trade Agreement. In the capital, he was considered a player, and a skilled one at that. Charming, courtly, low-key — on his wall hangs Lincoln's admonition that "persuasion, kind, unassuming persuasion, should ever be adopted" — Holmer came to the trade organization in 1996, near the eclipse of the noisy but brief Gingrich revolution. Brief, but enduring: the Gingrichian conservatives left Holmer with one lasting earful — PhRMA and its members would have to change their old practice of giving money to both political parties if it were to count on the GOP's aid in the future. It was a message that party hacks and honchos alike would hammer home to pharma executives again and again. As Jon Nicholson, the chairman of the Republican National Committee, baldly put it in a memo to the head of all brand-name companies in 1999, "We must keep our lines of communication open if we are to continue passing legislation that will benefit your industry." In the vernacular of an only slightly less elevated milieu, this might best be translated as "Yo, give it up, #!?@#I&#, or else!"

Over the next seven years, that is exactly what Holmer did. In election after election, and in legislative session after legislative session, he and the brand-name companies pumped huge amounts of cash into the Grand Old Party. Between 1999 and 2003, 79 percent of their $50 million in campaign contributions went to Republican causes and candidates. Individual members took up the call internally as well. In 2000 the CEO of Bristol-Myers Squibb sent urgent messages to all of his company's top managers to "donate the maximum" to the Bush campaign, $1,000 individually and $1,000 in their spouse's name; the company itself ponied up $2 million. In 2002, seeing that some form of prescription drug bill was inevitable, Holmer and his companies targeted $26 million for local congressional races. They also ratcheted up old-fashioned, buttonhole lobbying. By 2002 there were six pharma lobbyists for every sitting U.S. senator, a kind of political day care for potentially errant legislators.

To his delight, Alan Holmer found the Washington, D.C., so-cial climate enormously receptive to all this dough. Why, it was as if all of the antiquated reservations about taking money from big *anything* had simply vanished! The conservative think tanks that had once been the outsiders were now the insiders. They could be rallied to the intellectual support of the industry at the drop of a dime, mainly because most of them now received huge amounts of cash from the brand-name companies. Ditto the pa-tient groups and the cash cow, the American Association of Re-tired Persons, or AARP. All the "other side" had was that peevish Representative Henry Waxman and those unreasonable spoil-sport Naderites.

For pharma, the payoff was huge and swift. With each round of campaign contributions, each branch of the old buffering force — executive, legislative, and regulatory — was reshaped and re-spun in the industry's favor. In achieving this goal, Holmer was singularly focused on one mission: infuse the system with "mar-ket values" and a competitive ethos. There is, of course, noth-ing wrong with market values — in the market. But unlike Lew Engman, who had seen worth in the FDA's protective regula-tions, or Gerry Mossinghoff, who had seen his main mission as remaking pharma's connection to patients, Holmer understood that in permanently polarized D.C., using lobbying and money was about *preemptively* altering and reducing any form of regu-lation to the good of an abstract concept of the market.

That applied, too, at the state level. When governors began talking about laws to import cheaper medications from abroad, Holmer underwrote a huge campaign to warn consumers of the dangers of such drugs. (That there was almost no evidence to support this contention did not seem to matter.) Even for-eign governments got the treatment. When Canadian regulatory agencies looked to be clamping down on drug pricing, Holmer commissioned a special advertising and lobbying budget, tar-geted, it said, at nothing less than "changing the Canadian health care system." Even old pharma hands thought that was over the top. "Can you believe that?" said one of Pfizer's former lobbyists. "I would be embarrassed at that."

But shame, like equanimity, sincerity, and moderation, is not part of national political culture now, and whether one can blame Bill Clinton or George W. Bush remains unclear. What *is* clear is that the Holmer doctrine worked: Change the system. Get in early. And there was no better way than to get in early on the selection of a new FDA chief.

The pick of an FDA commissioner has always been political, and neither Democrats nor Republicans, let alone pharma, have ever quite mastered the art of getting exactly whom they wanted. David Kessler, Mr. Cigarettes Are Drugs, was an appointee of George the First. Mary Henney, who presided over more drug recalls than any agency chief in modern history, was a Clinton appointee. Neither proved particularly sympathetic to the industry. Holmer learned something from that: if you wanted to increase your odds of getting a decent candidate, you had to create the context. To do so, postelection 2000, he and his members drew up a list of the leading seventy-five contenders for the job, then circulated it, using the latest Internet technology, to the heads and VPs of his member companies, soliciting comments and getting consensus before the process began. To coordinate the effort, Holmer put a man named Bert Spilker in charge.

Almost immediately Spilker, a veteran pharma regulatory affairs expert, spotted trouble. The new Bush administration was moving quickly toward a candidate, Dr. Alastair Wood, and Wood was no friend of pharma. He was not exactly an enemy either. Wood is among the most respected clinical pharmacologists in the nation. He was the drug review editor for the *New England Journal of Medicine*, and he was a leading proponent of gene-driven drug development. But Wood had committed three primal offenses in the eyes of pharma. He had dared to cross swords with Pfizer in advisory committee meetings. Even worse, he had dared to call for the creation of an independent drug safety board, a reasonable enough notion to most human beings but one that sounded like "I eat Satan flakes for breakfast" to Holmer's CEOs. And Wood had spoken publicly about another heresy: perhaps, he said, it would be a good idea to wait for a while before doing DTC on new drugs. That did it for him. As Spilker recalls,

"When I got the list back from circulation among the members, there were exactly two names circled for elimination." One was Dr. Ray Woolsey, another highly respected clinical pharmacologist, who had already taken his name out of contention, and one was Alastair Wood.

Until then, the Wood nomination seemed a cinch. He had met not once, but many times with the White House personnel office, as well as with Scott McClellan, the president's communications chief, and Mark McClellan, Scott McClellan's brother and the head of the president's Council of Economic Advisers. "I had a strong sense that, if the president signs on, you've got the job," Wood recalls being told of the discussions. Many in the small but distinguished field of clinical pharmacology cheered.

The Holmer-Pfizer machine then kicked into high gear. First, it compiled a list of Wood's hundreds of published journal articles, underscoring the ones that advocated regulation and, in particular, the independent safety review board. The list found its way to an engaging writer on the predictably pro-pharma *National Review*, who promptly used the list to slam the candidate, likening him to David Kessler (the pre-DTC-loving Kessler, that is). In turn, Pfizer's PR department aggressively circulated the article. And Hank McKinnell, Pfizer's chief, may not have personally presented the administration with his objections, but he was and is the administration's closest pharma intimate, flying on cabinet-level trade and aid missions and sitting alongside the president at economic conferences. Not long after the borking had begun in earnest, Wood was informed that he was out. He says: "One of the lessons that came out of this for me is that people who had strong publishing records were easier to attack and dismiss, and how troubling that was."

All along, there had been someone pharma really wanted, but whose name they dared not utter: Dr. Les Crawford, then the deputy chief of the FDA. Crawford was a well-known entity. Industrious, experienced on both the food and drug sides, he had worked at the agency on and off for many years, and he had worked in the industry as well. He understood toxicology, and he was inclined toward the industry's view of how the agency should evaluate drugs. He was no industry hack, but he was hardly the forceful advocate for an independent drug safety board that Wood was. He believed that the agency should "manage" risk. "We shouldn't be averse to risk," he liked to declaim. "Risk is an integral part of life." As Spilker admitted, "The industry would be pleased if Les would become the commissioner." There was only one problem. Les was not a physician. Les was a veterinarian, and as Spilker well knew, that would never sell in the pedigree-conscious Senate, despite that august body's perennial need for rabies shots.

And so the administration picked one from its own loyal ranks: Dr. Mark McClellan. He was a nice enough fellow, but also someone with few publications and almost nothing on the record about drug regulation. It would be hard to bork him. One thing was known about McClellan: he was against importation of drugs from abroad. For Holmer et al., that was good enough. In fact, McClellan was perfect. The nomination sailed through, not least because the nation had by this time been without an FDA chief for almost three years.

Right away McClellan went on the warpath against imported drugs, the industry's number one economic issue and, in its view, a clear and present threat to the survival of the republic. He dispatched inspectors to U.S. postal centers and customs houses to document the extent of the problem, and pushed FDA publicists to woo reporters to write stories about the threat to public health of imports. Many newspapers bit, this despite the almost simultaneous publication of a study in the *New England Journal of Medicine* that concluded that inexpensive Canadian imports "posed no excess health risks for patients in the United States." Apparently McClellan did not have a subscription.

The new FDA chief then turned to the issue of drug promotion. There McClellan's priority was to change the FDA's image within the pharmaceuticals community, a novel use of government funds. Under him, the agency morphed from a tough, independent-minded regulatory body to a partner in nurturing pharmaceutical promotion. And so, on the January 2004 cover of *Medical Marketing and Media*, McClellan could be found with

Peter Pitts, his new public affairs director, alongside the headline "We won't bite." In an interview inside the magazine, Pitts
bragged about how he had welcomed visiting drug representatives, even offering to edit advertising and communication pro-
posals before the agency itself vetted them. Pitts and McClellan
then went on the pharmaceuticals speakers' circuits, appearing
at marketing confabs that promised to teach attendees things
like "how to push the promotional envelope."

In the rank and file of FDA staff, the McClellan effect was pronounced. Soon advocating the regulation of anything but the
most over-the-top and misleading drug promotion activity was
viewed, internally, as a career-killing move. The Division of
Drug Marketing, Advertising and Communications (DDMAC),
the tiny department charged with such regulation, grew rife with
institutional second-guessing. The consequence, as a congressional report would later find, was that in 2003 DDMAC issued
drug makers 75 percent fewer warning letters, its chief en-
forcement device, than it did during the last two years of the
Clinton administration. Even the pharmaceuticals trade press
was stunned by the change, noting in one headline that "Most
Medical Promotion Is Out of Sight of Regulators."

And then, in March 2004, the McClellan epoch ended as
abruptly as it had begun. McClellan took a job as the head of
Medicare, where, upon looking at the stunning cost of drugs for
that program, he promptly reversed himself on the issue of drug
imports. At the FDA, pharma got the man it really wanted all
along: Les Crawford. The hand of Holmer had prevailed.

And prevailed and prevailed. Indeed, one of the striking things
about the FDA was just how open it was to the industry and how
open it was about that openness. The half-open window of the
early 1990s had become a garage door, and a number of remarkable individuals were now driving through, looking for a career-
bumping burger and fries. Consider the strange case of Dan Troy,
who in 2001 became the FDA's chief counsel, every American's
legal insurer of FDA integrity.

When we last encountered Troy, of course, he was busily re-
crafting the legal basis for advertising just about anything to just

about anyone: tobacco, liquor, and, of course, DTC prescription drugs. And he was winning. Why, it was as if Troy had drunk from a secret elixir available only to members of his cherished Federalist Society, and then slipped a few milligrams of it into the drinking water of the federal appeals court: Troyism had become a growth industry in itself! And now came George W. Bush, who had brought with him no small contempt for regulation, restrictions, and, of course, plaintiffs' lawyers. Troy was well known by the president's chief adviser, Karl Rove; in 1995 Troy had successfully argued in front of the Supreme Court against then Governor Bush in a case involving racial gerrymandering that allegedly benefited Democrats. Not surprisingly, one of the new president's first appointments to the FDA was Troy. His brief: all legal-policy issues pertaining to FDA activities. It was a ballsy appointment, considering that Troy's firm had made more than $350,000 that year from one client, Pfizer. To avoid the inevitable hell to pay from Senator Edward Kennedy's review committee, the new president named Troy as a political appointee rather than as a nominee to the civil service, thereby circumventing any nasty public hearings.

There is nothing particularly unprecedented or tainted about naming someone with industry ties to a government counsel post, but there was something unprecedented in what Troy did not long after taking office (after one year — the legal minimum for taking any action involving a former client). In short, he sat down and met with attorneys for Pfizer and then filed an unsolicited friend-of-the-court brief in a case involving Zoloft and suicide. In it, Troy argued forcefully for the notion of "preemption" — that patients should not be allowed to sue drug makers for injury from their products because, he said, the FDA had established the drug's safety. If patients were allowed to sue, they might undermine the authority of the agency. He then went even further; along with lawyers at Justice, he argued that the threat of lawsuits by patients "can harm public health" by encouraging drug makers to withdraw products or issue new warnings that might emphasize risks and hence lead to "underutilization of beneficial treatments." Although this statement might seem amazing, especially to someone like Mark Miller, who believed his child very likely died because Pfizer did not emphasize the risks at all, such was the prevailing sentiment in the FDA's legal offices. That it was a dramatic departure from previous FDA opinions, which traditionally held that the agency merely established the "floor" of safety and that states could demand higher standards, did not seem to matter. Patients were preempted. Although Troy resigned in November 2004, the Troy doctrine persists, and has resulted in one case, involving a defective heart pump, being thrown out of court.

It was one thing to deal with electoral and regulatory politics, but, as Holmer well knew, it was quite another to deal with Congress, a mean dog to wrestle. Yet Holmer knew exactly where to throw the bait as it became clear, in 2003, that some form of the dreaded Medicare prescription drug bill would be passed. Holmer decided he could win on one count: populist inclinations against big government. As the organization had done in the early 1990s, when it campaigned against Bill and Hillary Clinton's health care plan, Holmer drafted two unlikely characters to make his case in the media: Harry and Louise, the smart-talkin' seniors on a mission to protect America from a government that seemed bent, in this case, on "getting into my medicine cabinet." Holmer spent millions on the campaign. Suddenly, the likable couple was in ads everywhere, recreating the same environment of fear and hysteria that had doomed other major health care legislation.

With the context of the debate now spun, Holmer turned to his main concern: governmental purchasing power. Almost every industrialized democracy — and not a few third world countries — used such power to wring out better prices for national health plans. They were a big reason drug prices were so high in the United States. The new Medicare bill held the prospect of the United States going the same way. Holmer, channeling his members' worst nightmares, hated the notion with a passion, and promptly put it in the center of his lobbying campaign. After a lengthy series of bills, amendments, House-Senate conferences, and rewrites, he and his allies, notably the AARP, prevailed. In

December 2003, the Medicare Prescription Drug Act became law. In it, governmental price wrangling was not just dropped, it was expressly banned.

To what extent was the Medicare bill and pharma's role in it something beyond the normal horse-trading that takes place on a daily basis in the nation's capital? No one really knows; the capital at present is an unfathomable brothel to all but the Reverends Rove and Cheney. But John Iglehart, the editor of the influential journal *Health Policy* and one of the more respected, even-tempered observers of pharma power, detects a clear and troubling thrust. "The contributions of pharmaceutical manufacturers that provide financial assistance to candidates through their political action committees, soft-money contributions that support advertising designed to influence policy, and other efforts add up to one of Washington's most elaborate advocacy strategies," he writes. "These efforts reinforced the natural instinct of most Republicans (and more than a few Democrats) to accommodate the interests of private enterprise when making policy, if at all possible."

Pharmaceutical money, "natural instinct," accommodation, Republicans, Democrats, the FDA: what, exactly, remains of the old, independent buffering force? It is, to reiterate the wisdom of *Medical Marketing and Media*, totally "out of sight." And mind.

At least until lately . . . Lately, Americans have started to ask The Question: What happens when money, shifting social currents, money, advertising, money, political accommodation, money, medical hubris, money, managed care, and, you get it, seem to all go to the good of one industry? The Question burps out another: Will success spoil pharma itself? It remains in our best interest to preserve the industry's better angels; that's where the great drugs *can* come from. The answer is still unclear. Consider, for example, the case of Merck.

On November 18, 2004, Americans were treated to a rare spectacle involving Merck, that awesome temple of pharmaceutical science. Ray Gilmartin, the company's chief executive, was forced to testify in front of a Senate committee investigating the recall of the company's pain pill Vioxx. Many hoped for a great

TV moment, perhaps à la the infamous 1995 testimony ("I do not believe that nicotine is addictive") by tobacco executives. Certainly the daggers were out for Gilmartin, wielded both by the usual suspects (Nader, Waxman, and the other "spoilers") and by the more aggressive elements of the investor-analyst community, who had long felt that the quiet Gilmartin, with his basset hound eyes, played his cards just a little too close to the vest for their speculating ways. The stock price had plummeted after Merck recalled Vioxx.

But Gilmartin surprised everyone. He came to the hearings alone, without the usual swarm of corporate attorneys that cheapen such affairs. Patiently, ploddingly, he led the dolts on the dais through Merck's thinking process on Vioxx: The company had acted ethically. There was no compelling reason to withdraw the drug until September 30, 2004, he said, when a new trial showed that Vioxx was linked to a doubling of risk for heart failure in some patients. Why, even my wife took it until then, Gilmartin revealed. It was a masterly corporate perp walk, performed perfectly, and perhaps genuinely, for a nation that wanted to believe that money and medicine could coexist without killing the patient. In the halls of pharma everywhere — but mainly in its capital, New Jersey — rose a sigh of great relief. Everyone went out for a steak and a bottle of red.

Outside the echo chamber of Washington, D.C., and pharma offices, however, new forces were gathering — and they were not so reassuring. One consisted of states' attorneys general, who began to pick up the federal government's dropped ball on pharma oversight. Perhaps the most aggressive of these reformers — if one was a pharma attorney, the phrase was "the biggest asshole" — was Eliot Spitzer, the attorney general of the state of New York. Spitzer had been fighting a variety of white-collar shenanigans when, in 2004, he filed suit against Glaxo for suppressing negative data on Paxil. In doing so, Spitzer devised a novel legal strategy that had not yet occurred to Dan Troy. As Spitzer saw it, it was a case of *fraud* if a drug maker does not tell physicians about trials of a medication that raise concerns about safety. As he told the *New York Times*, "I'm certainly not the person to determine whether Paxil is appropriate or not for any given person, but what I can do is ensure the information to doctors is fair and complete so that those equipped to make this determination can do so." He wanted a sizable chunk of Glaxo's $3 billion in annual Paxil sales to do so.

In other states, pharma was under siege by a new generation of corporate whistleblowers and U.S. attorneys. The most spectacular was a case initiated by David Franklin, the medical affairs detailer who had first detected something unethical in Tony Wild and Parke-Davis's off-label marketing of the epilepsy drug Neurontin in the mid-1990s ("Neurontin for pain . . . Neurontin for everything"!). In 2002, Franklin had joined with the U.S. attorney in Boston to sue Pfizer, which had acquired Parke-Davis, for illegal and fraudulent promotion of drugs, many of which had been paid for by Medicaid and other public agencies. In May 2004, Pfizer pleaded guilty and agreed to pay $430 million in penalties. The whistleblower tactic is now being imitated around the country, fueled in no small part by ambitious prosecutors and a small provision in the whistleblower statutes that allow informants to share in the massive settlements. Schering-Plough has since ponied up $350 million. Tap Pharmaceuticals: $875 million. Bayer: $257 million. And Merck, for abusing its Merck-Medco database: $30 million. Sometime soon, there will be hell to pay in shareholder meetings.

And there were the trial lawyers, who were now partying over the creation of a whole new arena of combat and lucre. Around the country, huge confabs of them gathered in giant meeting places — the Pasadena Civic Auditorium was one — to discuss strategy for class-action suits against Pfizer, Merck, Glaxo, and Schering. The scenarios at such shindigs were so optimistic that the subject most often discussed was not the verity of the cases or the chance of success, but which group of attorneys would take on what region of the country in the search for plaintiffs. Celebrity lawyers like the late Johnnie Cochran, of O.J. fame, made the pilgrimage to conferences with such go-ahead names as "Mass Torts Made Perfect!" Sophisticated Internet technologies were deployed to find more clients. By 2003, some 8,700 people had sued Pfizer for damages over Rezulin alone, with 32,000 possible plaintiffs waiting in the wings. Bayer faced at least 8,600 claimants over the recalled statin Baycol. Wyeth, already beleaguered, was looking at another 90,000 additional victims of Redux. In 2005 (at the time of this writing), Merck's Vioxx liability was so huge as to elude any reality-based estimate.

And if many Americans were still willing to give pharma the *general* benefit of the doubt, when it came to the issue of pricing, the PR battle was all but lost. On that count, no one was buying the now nauseating line that high prices were simply a reflection of the high cost of developing new drugs. A Harris poll showed that a higher percentage of those asked about the issue believed that the real culprit was greed. One consequence: more and more Joe Average seniors simply blew off the law and went north to Canada or south to Mexico to get their Lipitor. There were even special travel agencies and buying clubs set up to help budget-minded elders do so. Worse still, the bad attitude was percolating down to the next generation. As John Landis, a senior vice president for pharmaceutical sciences at Schering-Plough, related a recent experience to the *New York Times*'s Gardiner Harris, "You would think that a party with their wives would be a friendly, safe gathering. But the conversation quickly got around to why the costs of medications are so high, why does the drug industry spend so much on marketing, and why is there greater access to medicines outside the United States. They were unconvinced. So finally I had to say, 'Sooo, how about that football game?'" Even the ex–Merck executive Roy Vagelos, Gilmartin's predecessor, peeped his head out of retirement to decry the "exorbitant" prices. "This industry delivered miracles, and now they're throwing it all away," he fumed of his successors. "They just don't get it."

And how about the next generation of drugs, drugs that are true and safe breakthroughs and which, when all is said and done, would assure the betterment of human health? Where were they? For a decade, pharma had been tacitly suggesting to the public a deal: if American consumers could tolerate the hideous prices for chronic disease drugs *just a little longer*, the industry would soon be able to proffer a new generation of great drugs for both acute and noncurable diseases. But such has simply not happened. True, there have been a few breakthroughs in cancer therapies, but they were hardly the medicines the industry had promised for wide application. Between 1998 and 2003, the number of newly introduced compounds shrank dramatically, from fifty-three to seventeen. The decrease had nothing to do with the usual scapegoat, the FDA. The real reason, slowly acknowledged in private and then in public: the very mergers that were supposed to have helped the companies carve out even greater global share. These mergers instead turned out to be team-wrecking, momentum-slowing, lab-shattering experiences in most big companies, GlaxoSmithKline chief among them. There, the cupboards were bare. Lab heads are at odds, and such high-tech industry cure-alls as high-throughput screening — computerized drug candidate testing — have been major and costly disappointments.

Yet instead of focusing on this core of issues, the industry has gone into reengineering mode. Expensive "big think" consultants are drafted by the score. Internal "change initiatives," led by overpaid managerial whizfolk, abound. Paralysis reigns. A rare inside view of the whole scene was rendered in late 2003, by Maryann Gallivan, a vice president in global life-sciences investing at the financial giant Cap Gemini Ernst and Young. Because Gallivan splits her time between monitoring sales and science initiatives, she occasionally gets an insight into just how slow the process for true breakthrough drugs has become. Speaking to a select group of the United Kingdom's biggest pharma executives, Gallivan was asked how hard it was to track research and development trends these days. "Oh," Gallivan replied. "It's not hard at all. I go away from R&D for a couple of years to work on sales. When I come back, I don't have much to catch up on."

And more and more, a breed of executives who had for long successfully shielded themselves from criticism by invoking overregulation began to look within. It was not pretty. The incredibly low return on research and development investment? The near mythical $800 million price tag for developing new drugs? It was their own fault. They were choosing targets badly. "Productivity," as AstraZeneca's John Symonds admitted to a small group of fellow executives, "is not something that this industry has been known for [during] the past fifteen years."

By late 2004, blockbusterism, the jumbo golden Rx goose, seemed to have laid its last egg. There were just so many drugs that one could sell to mass audiences, without, of course, either getting burned by off-label injuries or by spending so much on DTC that it wrecked profit-and-loss statements. And anyway, the blockbuster approach, as Dr. Duncan Moore, a biochemist with Morgan Stanley, put it, was based on a historical anomaly. "From about 1991 to 1996, we had a period of disequilibrium in this industry," he explained. Regulators were not ready for the onslaught of new, me-too drugs, despite the fact that they were relatively easy to develop, and managed care, willing to do about anything except pay for more expensive doctors' office visits and procedures, gave many such drugs a blank check. "During that period," Moore said, "the default went to the more expensive option. Not now."

5

Independence for Generation Rx

What Can Be Done

THERE IS A WAY BACK to independence. It is not an easy way, and it is not a short path. But it is a fair one, I hope, with demands on everyone, from pharma to patient.

First comes the physician, who remains our front-line pharma buffer. But what do we know about our doctors, and what should we expect from them when it comes to "relations" with the industry? Robert Goodman, an internist and assistant professor of clinical medicine at Columbia University, has been looking hard at that question for years now, ever since he was a med student in the 1980s, when he grew uneasy eating pizzas provided gratis by drug detailers. By the late 1990s, Goodman had grown convinced, through a wide range of published research, that all pharma freebies — from mugs and notepads to expensive dinners and trips — should be spurned. All physicians should refuse them. He started a one-man organization, No Free Lunch, to spread the message. On his Web site he offers "pen amnesty" and a free No Free Lunch pen to physicians who send in their drug-company swag. He also uses the site to get fellow doctors to take what he calls "The Pledge" — a vow not to accept any such perks in the future.

While only three hundred or so have officially signed on, Goodman's effort has helped to congeal a fast-growing, if still small, movement among medical students and their professors to educate young doctors about the extent and practice of medical marketing. (And if the vitriol sent in by opposing physicians is any indication, he has hit a raw nerve among the established medical class as well.) On the surface, the movement calls to mind the med students of the late 1960s and 1970s, who saw putting limits on pharma influence as part of a greater skein of social justice. Today's reformers are largely motivated by something more pragmatic; theirs are ethical and professional concerns aimed at salvaging the reputation of medicine by putting more distance between physicians — both academicians and practitioners — and pharmaceutical power.

The flash point for such efforts is at the University of California, San Francisco (UCSF), which was embarrassed not long ago by a number of publicized cases in which unflattering clinical trial results were suppressed to please pharma sponsors. There, one approach to limit pharma influence might involve the creation of an independent, not-for-profit intermediary body responsible for all interactions between physician-scientists and companies. Such was the tack suggested by Dr. Mary-Margaret Chren some ten years ago. Chren is a dermatologist who serves on the financial sponsorship review committee at UCSF. While her proposal was ignored at first, the time may be ripe for resuscitation. Disclosure and transparency are increasingly key issues, both ethically and pragmatically, she argues. "Our system would never tolerate judges taking money from those that they judge, yet for some reason this doesn't apply in medicine," she told the *British Medical Journal* recently. "Doctors feel they should have complete freedom with no protection from potentially compromising relationships." Under a report commissioned by UCSF's medical school dean in 2002, the school headed toward a ban on free lunches sponsored by pharmaceutical firms and an end to direct sponsorship of all educational events on campus. There are also moves to limit the largely unrestricted access by drug reps to physicians and, often, to patients. Again, students are providing much of the push. The biggest comes from the 30,000-member American Medical Student Association. In a campaign dubbed PharmFree, med students are asked to sign what the group calls the "model oath for the new physician." Its core: "I will make medical decisions . . . free from the influence of advertising or promotion. I will not accept money, gifts, or hospitality that will create a conflict of interest in my education, practice, teaching, or research."

Should these students ever be taken seriously — and there are growing signs that they are — their pledge would radically reshape physician continuing medical education, or CME. Pharma, as we have seen, currently underwrites nearly 90 percent of all such education, and any limits on what has come to be regarded as a kind of professional entitlement will face huge institutional opposition, particularly from older physicians who take enormous umbrage at any suggestion that such perks lead to poor treatment decisions. After all, they ask, Where will the money come from if not from pharma? Drummond Rennie, a deputy editor of the *Journal of the American Medical Association* and a professor of medicine at UCSF, has little use for such arguments. "That . . . presupposes that some of the most well-off in our society can't afford to pay for their own lunches, their education, or their conference. But guess what: all sorts of poorer people pay every step of the way. No one is handing out money to them. When I hear doctors crying poverty . . . and an inability to pay for their education, I feel ashamed of my profession." William Vodra, a one-time FDA attorney and now one of the nation's leading pharmaceutical legal hands, puts it bluntly: "Can you think of any other profession that actually expects to have its continuing education for free?"

While we are on the subject of physician integrity, I have another radical suggestion: How about a requirement for a "physician history" to go along with every request for a patient history? Such a document, attached to the clipboard carrying the obligatory patient bio, would answer key questions, ranging from the perfunctory — physician's name, education, latest CME courses, publications, awards — as well as the doctor's significant financial relationships with pharma and pharma-connected groups, including consulting fees, speaking fees, clinical-trial investigator payments, stock and equity positions. There are a number of less extreme permutations, of course, including one that would simply state the relationship without the amount of money involved. That way the patient is informed of the extent of the unseen presence in the exam room without violating the doctor's financial privacy. Yet any such attempt will likely be met with hostility by the AMA, which has long opposed even the most mundane disclosure measures. Fortunately, more and more state legislatures simply don't care about the AMA's position. They have successfully enacted laws requiring that physicians, for example, reveal malpractice settlements — one measure of physician performance. To restore fully patient-physician trust, we must extend that transparency even further. Being independent from pharmaceutical influence matters.

Now that the AMA has a surveillance camera trained on my house, let us turn to pharma itself. What can we do to make the industry more responsible? The answer, bane to every pharma-bankrolled congressman and think tank, is more independent regulation. By this I mean the kind of regulation that even conservatives once acknowledged was not only acceptable, but also healthy (before, that is, conservatives like Lew Engman were replaced by conservatives like Gerry Mossinghoff and Alan Holmer). First and foremost, we must return the FDA to its roots. Its job, mandated by law, is to *regulate an industry*, not to be some skanky "proactive partner" with that industry. And to do that, we must first end — or at least deeply modify — the agency's client-type relationship with pharmaceutical companies.

To do *that*, we must take a few hard initial steps. First, if we want a more independent FDA, free from the monkey business that has so enraged Americans over the past few years, we must be willing to spend some money, and that will likely be somewhere around $1 billion a year. That is the amount pharma now pays in "fees" to get products reviewed in a timely fashion through PDUFA, the Prescription Drug User Fee Act. Speaking of PDUFA: it should not be renewed. That will help put an end to the sweatshop environment in the agency, and take away any "legitimate" pressure to hurry through new drugs. Truly urgent new compounds — for cancer — can be shepherded through a division focused on expanded investigational drug trials. The agency should also spend more money on two new surveillance systems for adverse effects. One would focus on the liver, the other on birth defects. These are difficult but clearly wide-ranging public health concerns that only a combination of government clout and resources can sustain for the long, trial-and-error period required. More money to watch for liver damage and birth defects: It is hard to imagine these would fail to pass muster in man-in-the-street tests, both red and blue streets.

Money is not the only thing required to set the agency right. New legislation must be passed as well (although who would have the moxie and will to spearhead it is unclear). Such legislation would confer specific new powers on the FDA, powers most Americans probably think it already has but which it doesn't. For example, the agency must establish and fund a separate drug safety unit, one independent of the drug review division; such would help put an end to the enabling culture that created the Vioxx and Paxil messes. This is the same measure that Alastair Wood was so viciously hammered for when nominated to head the agency four years ago, but which now finds favor in such strange regions as that of Republican Senator Charles Grassley. That same legislation should also grant the FDA the power to *require* Phase Four, or postmarketing, safety trials. Such studies are currently routinely requested as a condition of approval — and then promptly ignored by nearly every major drug maker. The agency must also be empowered to establish a comprehensive national clinical trial registry, so that regulators and clinicians can independently assess pharma claims of safety and efficacy; such was one of the many lessons of SSRIs and children. And it must be able to require so-called head-to-head trials — trials that establish the superiority of a new compound over an existing compound, not simply a 5 percent improvement over a sugar pill. Lastly, to ensure that Dan Troy, the Federalist Society, and law firms for the broadcast industry have something to litigate against for the next few years, the FDA should request a voluntary hold on DTC ads for every new drug it approves; under this guidance, DTC — including disease awareness — for any new drug product should wait two years before commencing the usual ask-your-doctor-now campaign. The money pharma would save would allow it to reduce prices, do better clinical studies, and fund more meaningful research.

As we enter what the D.C. think tanks will likely label as "a new era of Stalinist regulation," let us turn to the patent office. Yes, the patent office, the chug-chug little agency that initiated the new era. Here is what its new mantra should be: patents on drugs should be given only to compounds that are *better* than existing compounds, not just better than a placebo. Such was Senator Kefauver's thinking on the matter as far back as the early 1960s, and it still makes sense today. To draft such guidelines, the patent office should recruit Gerry Mossinghoff, who could do a lot to nudge and coax the initiative in the right direction while maintaining his éminence-grise status across the river in Alexandria and perhaps curbing a little of his own pharma karma. The patent office should also be required to use a new generation of patent software (there is a remarkable one by the software giant SAS) to do deeper research into which supposed drug innovations are really novel and which are simply semantic license. For example, almost every single time-release technology used today to justify a new patent for an existing drug (and so ratchet up its price) is in reality an old technology that does nothing but increase the overall drug load on the human body. New software can help the patent office separate the wheat from the chaff, with the citizen — and not just the patent applicant — in mind. What a concept.

And what of Congress itself? Remember, Congress is the only entity to possess the subpoena power needed to force pharma to produce all documents. That's increasingly important during those times when the industry fails to disclose everything to the FDA and it comes back to bite us on the collective COX-2 inhibitor. Yet the use of congressional power over the industry has been inconsistent, disorganized, and often irresponsible, both on the right and left. It has been lorded over long enough by Henry Waxman, who is good at playing the hysteria card, and Orrin

Hatch, who tries to trump him with the "let's keep America competitive" card. Both have their strengths, but both also hold views that are out of touch with Americans' constantly evolving attitudes and expectations about pharma and government. Who, exactly, is independent and tough-minded enough to take their places is anyone's guess, particularly in a culture where the default is increasingly owned and operated by pharma. To wit, the new CEO of the trade organization PhRMA (the new Alan Holmer) is none other than Billy Tauzin, only a year or so ago the head of the Senate Commerce Committee and the main architect of the no-negotiating clause in the new Medicare Prescription Drug law.

What can be done to make pharma itself better and safer?

At the dawn of the modern pharma era, there was one crucial player who never quite got onto the proverbial playing field: the *independent* clinical pharmacologist. Clinical pharmacologists study how drugs work in a medical, rather than experimental, setting. The great heyday of clinical pharmacology took place in the early 1960s, when drug efficacy was first mandated and medical institutions took up the cause with great passion and idealism. Yet the professionalization of clinical pharmacology never gained firm footing, either in the academy or in private practice. Medical schools found the discipline hard to fathom, particularly in an era of extreme specialization. If you graduated someone as a clinical pharmacologist and he did not go to work for a drug company, well, for whom would he work? Physicians were more pragmatic, asking simply: What was the billing code? The result was that by the 1990s clinical pharmacology, once the great hope for independent drug evaluation, had waned. In 2003, the average medical student got one class on the subject during her entire training. That course is usually taught by a Ph.D. whose main experience is with rats, not humans. This state of affairs is a good one if you are a rat seeking appropriate pharmaceutical care, but not so good if you aren't.

Art Atkinson, the senior adviser at the NIH's Clinical Center, has been thinking about the gap between drug lab knowledge and physician knowledge for a long time. He is an old hand in the arena of clinical pharmacology and in the 1970s made a singular contribution that affects many patients today. Atkinson's idea was to require hospital blood labs to collect and analyze blood samples of patients who were taking the heart drug digoxin, which can be highly toxic. This practice he dubbed "therapeutic drug monitoring." The process helps clinicians see exactly how a given drug concentrates in various subpopulations. That, in turn, gives hospitals better and more precise guidelines for the safe and effective use of the drug. In short, doctors don't poison as many people by overreliance on pharma's often unrealistic (too high) dosage regimens. It is a relatively inexpensive measure that has been widely embraced by the medical community and hospitals around the world.

Atkinson has another idea now, one designed to unblock the information flow from lab tests to hospital decision makers. It sounds like a no-brainer, which is what many good ideas sound like when they are freed from the bullshit-athon of formal medical policy discourse. The logjam, says Atkinson, *speaking as a private individual and not as the powerful head of a giant NIH department,* lies in every major and most small hospitals' pharmacy and therapeutics, or "P&T," committees. Such committees are charged with monitoring new and old drugs, deciding what to add to hospital formularies, and with monitoring medication usage patterns. They are the drug czars of the hospital. As Atkinson sees it, the opportunity to chair such a committee should be a highly sought-after opportunity. Yet it is not. Why? Because P&Ts are not taken seriously, he says. And why is that? Because the Joint Commission on Accreditation of Hospitals, the private agency that gives its influential seal of approval to institutions, does not require that P&T committees sit as formally constituted bodies. The rationale is that such a requirement would make the committee too rigid.

But in almost any complicated organization — and hospitals are extremely complicated — committees that are essentially *ad hoc* often become second-rate. "It ends up being [chaired by] someone who is very junior who *has* to do it rather than people who are qualified to do it," Atkinson says. And that means that the collectors and evaluators of drug information for many huge health systems end up with lots of data and little in the way of wisdom. Why, for instance, wasn't Vioxx delisted from formularies until Merck withdrew it? The answer now lies on the conscience of many lackluster P&T committee chairpeople, who should give Atkinson's ideas a little more time — or turn the responsibility over to those who take the task seriously.

Such ideas do not get a huge amount of attention for another reason: they don't involve blaming it all on pharma, and that's no fun. I'll get to the fun soon enough, but first let's visit one other idea that will require use of your higher cognitive functions. The idea comes from Alastair Wood, one of the leading clinical pharmacologists of our age, and from a number of his colleagues in the field. Recall that it was Wood who was blackballed by Pfizer and its cohorts when his name was circulated for nomination to head the FDA a few years ago. Still the drug review editor for the *New England Journal of Medicine*, Wood has since taken up the subject of pharmacogenetics with a vengeance. Pharmacogenetics is the study of how genes — both in individuals and in populations — affect the way the human body metabolizes, distributes, and gets rid of various drugs. Wood now views pharmacogenetics as nothing less than the future of clinical pharmacology and big pharma as well. The reason for his passion on the subject is deceptively simple. As he tells it, the discipline holds the prospect of answering the primary question: "Does the drug work well enough to justify the bet?"

There are already early examples of how pharmacogenetics would change and improve medicine. Consider the growing work on the cytochrome P450 family of drug-processing liver enzymes that we visited earlier. Recall that different populations possess genetic traits that tweak the way some drugs are metabolized by 450. Recall also that some drugs tweak 450 itself. Some drugs induce the body to produce more of the enzyme, meaning that the effect of the drug may be shorter and more intense, while other drugs repress 450, causing the drug (or others in competition for metabolism) to stay in the body for longer periods of time. All of this is governed by genetic variants, usually involving many genes.

Genes, then, matter enormously — and sometimes can spell the difference between life and death — when certain drugs are used, and pharmacogenetics has a keen potential for ferreting out that crucial difference. Writing in the *New England Journal of Medicine* not long ago, William E. Evans and Howard L. McLeod predicted that the discipline will "yield a powerful set of molecular diagnostic methods that will become routine tools with which clinicians will select medications and drug doses for individual patients." As a result, "It may be possible to collect a single blood sample from a patient. Submit [it] . . . for analysis of a panel of genotypes, and test for those that are important determinants of drug disposition and effects." (Roche, Irwin Lerner's old company, has already made a small step in this direction, having developed a crude test, approved by the FDA in 2005, for certain P450 traits in patients.)

As Wood sees it, pharmacogenetics could not only revolutionize pharmacology and everyday medical practice, it could also deeply alter clinical trials, making them safer and more reliable. "It would be possible to genotype in trials who was a responder [in terms, say, of P450] and who was a nonresponder," he says. "By doing that, it would allow for early identification of those subjects who would overrespond or underrespond to any given regimen." That would make it possible to weed out patients who would be overly vulnerable to new agents — perhaps as was young Tracy Johnson in Lilly's trial for the new antidepressant Cymbalta — and, on the other hand, to test more toxic drugs on people with the genetic ability to handle them.

Yet for pharmacogenetics to fulfill its potential will take a huge investment in basic science. The human genome is made up of 1.4 million single nucleotide polymorphisms, and about 60,000 of those variants sit in the so-called coding region of genes, which translates into a huge diversity of multigene drug filters or prisms. If pharma is not wont to fund such an endeavor, who will take the plunge? One way of getting the money would be to reassess the priorities of the NIH, perhaps channeling some

taxpayer dollars away from programs that involve new compounds and instead target the human genome. The NIH started
such an effort in 2000, when its Pharmacogenetics Research Network began funding a series of projects to assemble, analyze, and
disseminate all available knowledge about how genetic varia-
tions in individuals contribute to differences in reactions to
drugs. One fruit of the effort is Stanford University's PharmGKB
network, which allows anyone interested to search an extensive
database for drug-gene information.

One doesn't have to use one's imagination to understand exactly how such data could affect individual patients. Dr. David
Flockhart, a pioneer in gene-drug interactions, has already blazed
that trail. Under the rubric of "rational prescribing," Flockhart
has compiled a list of known gene-based drug interactions involving a key liver enzyme system and has distributed that list
via pocket-sized cards now carried by hundreds of thousands of
physicians. It is already changing and improving patient care.
His Web site, Drug-Interactions.com, is visited by 10,000 physicians and scientists a month from around the world. Such is one
very American response to the problem of separating pharma
power from individual health decisions.

Ivan Illich, the prickly philosopher whose anti–medical establishment writings so inspired the originators of today's DTC advertising binge, may well be chuckling at all of this from heav-
enly realms. Illich died of cancer in 2002, a cancer he steadfastly
refused to treat with surgery, which, he was told, might render
him unable to hear or speak. Speech is not something anyone
wants to lose, especially a philosopher, whose stock in trade depends on it. So Illich quietly treated the pain of his neoplasm
with . . . opium. "One of the great traditional poisons," he called
it in an interview a few years before his passing.

It was completely in keeping with the views he had laid down
in *Medical Nemesis* almost thirty years ago. As Illich saw it, re-
sisting standardized treatment was all about reclaiming one's
medical identity — about picking one's own poisons and enduring, enduring, enduring. As he told the former California gover-

nor Jerry Brown, an intimate, "Yes, we suffer pain, we become ill, we die. But we also hope, laugh, celebrate; we know the joy of caring for one another; often we are healed and we recover by many means. We do not have to pursue the flattening-out of human experience. I invite all to shift their gaze, their thoughts, from worrying about health care to cultivating the art of living. And, today with equal importance, the art of suffering, the art of dying."

Few of us today, myself included, possess that stoic bent; fewer still the time, energy, and intellectual focus to spend on reclaiming something as amorphous as one's own "individual medical identity." We are not a society of philosophers; we are a society of producers and consumers. We are busy. We want to live, not die with a grapefruit-sized neoplasm on our face, as did Illich. We don't see pain and suffering as particularly inevitable or ennobling or even natural; we don't want to limp if we can still run.

The principal forces that have so deeply pharmaceuticalized American life are hardly likely to abate anytime soon. Managed care over the next decades will continue to depend heavily upon pills as a proxy for physician care. Cost-conscious employers and insurers will make sure of that. As will Wall Street — particularly as baby boomers begin to cash in their retirement funds, which have been floating on that nice, easy cushion of double-digit pharmaceutical company returns for two decades. The average pharma CEO will feel the heat and continue to do what he has been doing, only faster.

Yet there is a sliver of Illich's uncomfortable wisdom that might go a long way toward making prescription drugs safer, sounder, more rational, and *less compelling as a consumer product*. It is the notion of independence — independence in the main institutions and human attitudes that buffer our bodies and souls from pure pharmaceutical capitalism. This is not to say that we should not also look long and hard at the so-called meta-issues — the "shoulds." Should drug companies be allowed to advertise at all? Should we use government power to break up pharmaceutical monopolies? It is to say that, in the meantime, we might look to what *can* be done.

One question almost never asked in public debate about pharma is: How can we as individuals cut down on our own use of prescription drugs? The reticence is both understandable and maddening. The understandable: I once asked a top executive at the NIH whether anyone was studying the relationship between pharmaceutical harm and class. Do poor people, who get less medical oversight, tend to get hurt by prescription drugs more often than those who are better off? The answer, spoken *sotto voce*: "No one here is studying that, because all of the focus is on the fact that poor people have poor access to medicines. So the focus is on getting them better access to prescription drugs." Yes, of course.

But there is a maddening logic as well, and too often it prevails. Any insinuation that patients should self-regulate is either branded as unethical or as stigmatizing the sufferer. How, after all, can we live in such a compelling health-consumer society and expect anyone to say no to prescription drugs? True, people do it all the time; that is what "noncompliance" is, among other things. But simple noncompliance is a deadly gambit. There has to be a better way.

One route might be for patients to stop thinking of themselves as consumers, as buyers of health. Instead, we might think of ourselves as patients and focus on everything that goes into being a patient. Yet this is not the sole prescription for our woes, so before every patient advocacy group gets its collective shorts in a knot, read on.

First remember that yesterday's patient was transformed into today's "health care consumer" by a wide range of societal, economic, business, and political trends, from managed care to marketing to workplace and family demands to contemporary self-improvement culture. The result is a person with medical needs who wants to act as if he is not going to the doctor but rather to the mall. We want choices and to be consulted on those choices all along the way. And we want it all now. There's nothing wrong with patient empowerment, of course, and who doesn't say good riddance to the days of the "It's complicated — just take the meds, think about the surgery, and leave it up to me" doctor of yore? But truth be told, particularly when it comes to chronic diseases, there's another confession most of us need to make: America has become a nation of (big) half-asses, more in search of a compliant fellow to cosign our condition — and the pills that go with it — than someone who really wants to treat it in a sustained and serious fashion.

In fairness to physicians, we must as patients toughen up — toughen up our minds and our bodies. First, The body: if you want to pharmaproof yourself, or at least minimize your exposure to pharmaceutical risk, get a healthy life. Oh, sure, it's hard not to hoover down that trough of nightly Cheetos. After all, you deserve it! But maybe if you skipped the midnight snack, you wouldn't need the Ambien to get some sleep, or the Nexium for your bogus GERD. And you might actually have time to get some exercise. That does not mean that you should stop taking drugs that you really need — but it does mean that you've got to get involved in your care. And you do not need a pharma Web site to help you with that, despite what Pfizer might tell you. You can start with an honest, uncomfortable but pointed conversation with your physician about the drugs you are on. If you are dealing with an elderly parent, make an appointment and bring in the bottles of all the drugs he is currently taking. Insist that the physician evaluate the overall drug load. At the very least, have him check it against the Beers List (http://www.dcri.duke.edu/ccge/curtis/beers.html) of inappropriate drugs for the elderly.

Next, the mind: Stop with the consumer experimentation thing. When you think about drugs, recite these mantras: Drugs are poisons — useful poisons but poisons nonetheless. Every time you use one you also "use" one or more vital organs to process it. If it is a new drug, you are a test subject. If it is a clinical trial, *you are part of a human experiment.* Say it. Say it again. This statement serves as your counterprogramming to pharma's powerful billion-dollar programming. It's a small start, but it is a start.

It would be a hard heart, of course, that held that all sufferers of chronic disease should simply get tough, but it would be a soft head that turned away from the overwhelming data that show that Americans, more than any other nationality, are killing themselves with food, TV, and cigarettes. Prescription drugs have become a way of delaying premature death without dealing with the underlying soul and body sickness of modern life and modern life choices. This is complicated by the fact that while pharma will always be with us, deep down inside, Americans still don't fathom that pharma's principal allegiances are not to God, nature, and man, but to science, markets, and mammon. *It depends on us.*

The traditional liberal response is to say that we do not invest enough in wellness programs and preventive medicine. That may be true, but if one really wants to talk about wellness, the hidden issue here is class. It's the poor who don't have access to preventive medicine, to good prenatal care, to good nutrition and ample recreation. They don't even have the language to access it. Not the middle class. They've got it — they just don't use it. And why is that? They are simply too busy working and consuming. The answer for them is not a new wellness program, but it may lie in a deeper, more honest examination of modern work, school, and family life and its costs as well as its benefits. Physicians as well might take the little time they do have with patients to ask not what is wrong, but, what do you do? Occupational health: what a concept.

Here we actually have some wisdom from history, and it might pay for patients, physicians, and the government to heed it. The time is the Renaissance, the place northern Italy. Renaissance Italy posed, in some ways, many of the same health challenges that modern America does. It was a time and place where larger numbers of urban people (certainly not the high percentages of today, but larger numbers nonetheless) were confronted with relative caloric abundance. It was also a time of remarkable occupational opportunity and change. As cities grew under the enlightened beneficence of merchant kings, so did artisan classes and the concentrated working class to serve them. Jobs were plentiful, but they were also new to many from a one-time agrarian populace. Former breathers of fresh country air now worked in dusty, often chemically tainted indoor trades, as marble grinders, coppersmiths, plasterers, and printers. It is no surprise that the first proponent of occupational health, Bernardino Ramazzini, would arise out of such a dynamic work culture. Ramazzini's advice: "In work so taxing, moderation would be the best safeguard against these maladies, for men and women alike."

Occupational health, unfortunately, is not a top-line issue that late-twentieth- and early-twenty-first-century American politics has wanted to engage, despite enormous upheaval and stress in the modern workplace. The situation has largely been the inverse. Occupational health and safety have been whipping boys for antiregulatory politicians since the late 1970s, when the alleged brightest bulbs began to see things like the Occupational Safety and Health Act as a "threat to competitiveness," much to the delight of their big- and small-business donors. Organized labor too abused OSHA regulations to win turf wars with management over workplace control. As a result, OSHA is all but moribund; its list of publications and technical links reads as if most of the workforce were still in factories rather than on the computer or behind the wheel. Stress is not even part of the underfunded agency's lexicon. Occupational health is still not a serious player. Yet by not dealing with work and health in a steady, mature way — as do other industrialized democracies — we assume all the possible risks, and end up taking . . . more pills. At some point the productivity gains of an unhealthful workplace will be outstripped by the cost of treating the illnesses of the labor force with drugs that bring their own unknown woes. Nothing comes without a price.

That's why simply blaming Uncle Pharma just isn't enough anymore. We can't let the charming little bastard off the hook, and we have to go him one better. Americans and pharma must recognize the mutual intensity, emotionality, and deceptiveness of their codependence. We need to shed synergy. Only then can we honestly learn where our true interests converge and where they depart. The stakes are high. It's your money *and* your life.

A BRIEF GUIDE TO THE ART
OF TAKING PRESCRIPTION DRUGS

NOTES

INDEX

A Brief Guide to the Art
of Taking Prescription Drugs

Although there seems to be an unending gusher of health information in the United States, almost all of it is, in one way or another, the vehicle of a vested political or corporate interest. That does not mean that, *ipso facto,* such information is wrong, misleading, or bad; it just means that one should start with the presumption that a site for allergy sufferers, say, is probably funded by pharmaceutical companies, using studies developed and underwritten by drug companies, and, in general, telling patients the pharma side of the story first. Few sites say things like "assume that any new symptom you are having after starting a new drug may be caused by that drug," or "when adding a new drug to your regimen, see if it is possible to discontinue another drug."

One site that does voice such alternatives is maintained by Public Citizen (www.citizen.org), the single best resource for information on prescription drugs and how to take them responsibly and, as much as is possible, independently from the seductive buzz of pharma. The organization's two most helpful tools on this count are its annual guide, "Worst Pills," available for purchase via its own site (www.worstpills.org), and, at the same site for free, its "Ten Rules for Safer Drug Use." The "Ten Rules" page offers free access to an outstanding, simple worksheet that will help the average patient or patient advocate organize drug prescription information *before* a doctor appointment. Public Citizen also offers a number of ancillary guides, also free, ranging from "Diseases Caused by

Drugs" to "Facts and Myths About Generic Drugs" to "Cutting Your Prescription Drug Bill." It says something that the site is reviled in many pharma marketing circles, which almost never fault its facts, for its temerity to tell it like it is, using science, not spin.

The FDA's own site (www.fda.gov) is an enormous one, and confusing as well. Using the search engine will yield very specific information — for instance, the transcript of an advisory committee meeting about the safety of Paxil — and very general information about drug safety issues, some of which is worth reading. But a better site for detailed scholarly research about specific drugs is the Pub Med section of the National Library of Medicine (www.nlm .nih.gov); the search feature will give you abstracts and links to journals, where you can access (sometimes for free, often for a fee) the original full text. If you are not prepared to give yourself a mini–medical education, however, the site's clearly written "Medline Plus" and "NIH Senior" sections will prove less daunting.

On the subject of liver toxicity and the growing importance of genetic factors in that field, the highly readable site maintained by Indiana University's Dr. David A. Flockhart (http://medicine.iupui .edu/flockhart/), is a perfect primer, replete with a drug interactions page and pocket chart. Another outstanding resource on the liver and drugs in general is Howard J. Worman's *Liver Disorders Sourcebook* (Lowell House, 1999), and Dr. Worman's own site at Columbia University (http://cpmcnet.columbia.edu/dept/gi/disliv .html).

On the subject of children and psychiatric drugs, one book worth reading is Lawrence H. Diller's *Running on Ritalin* (Bantam, 1998), which is balanced, nuanced, and practical in a hardheaded way; much the same can be said for his Web site (www.docdiller.com). On the oft overlooked but crucial subject of dosage control, see Jay S. Cohen's *Overdose* (Tarcher-Putnam, 2001) for a reasoned, enlightening discussion and untainted wisdom. And see Cohen's site (www.medicationsense.com) for ongoing commentary and practical advice on topical issues.

What about polypharmacy, the soaring practice of multiple prescriptions for single and multiple diagnosis and arguably the looming time bomb of Generation Rx? There is little written about it in general. The best single source concerns geriatric polypharmacy, the now globally respected Beer's List of medications to avoid when treating patients over sixty-five. An outstanding and useful description of all Beer's List drugs can be found at the site of the Texas Association of Homes and Services for the Aging (www.tahsa .org/files%2FDDF%2Fmedbeer1.pdf). Print out two copies — one for your refrigerator and one for your doctor.

Notes

Introduction

page
1   "When a great profession": David Blumenthal, "Doctors and Drug Companies," *New England Journal of Medicine*, vol. 351, October 28, 2004, pp. 1885–90.
    "First there were French fries": Deborah Baldwin, "Medicine Cabinets: Walk Right In," *New York Times*, March 18, 2004, p. D1.
2   "He's obsessed with muscle power pills!": Ibid., p. D9.
    Over the past decade: "Kaiser Family Foundation Prescription Drug Trends — A Chartbook Update," November 2001, exhibit 16, p. 30. See also pp. 31–40. For 2004 figures, see "Kaiser Family Foundation Prescription Drug Trends Update," October 2004, p. 1.
    The cost per year?: National Center for Health Statistics, Centers for Disease Control, *Health, United States, 2004*, with chartbook on *Trends in the Health of Americans*, pp. 50–53.
    There's another number: Ibid.
3   On one day during the summer of 2004: See Gardiner Harris, "Anti-Depressants Seen as Effective for Adolescents," *New York Times*, June 2, 2004, p. 1. Also see Gardiner Harris, "Spitzer Sues a Drug Maker, Saying It Hid Negative Data," *New York Times*, June 3, 2004, p. 1.
8   more than 106,000 deaths: Jason Lazarou, Bruce H. Pomeranz, and Paul N. Corey, "Incidence of Adverse Drug Reactions in Hospitalized Patients: A Meta-analysis of Prospective Studies," *Journal of the American Medical Association* (*JAMA*), vol. 279, no. 15, April 15, 1998.

9   "The present drug regulatory system": John Abraham, "The
     Pharmaceutical Industry as Political Player," *Lancet*, vol. 360,
     2002, pp. 1498–1502, 1507.
     One more statistic: The National Institute for Health Care Man-
     agement Research and Educational Foundation, "Changing Pat-
     terns of Pharmaceutical Innovation," May 2002, p. 3.

1. Unbound

For the first section in this chapter, I interviewed nearly every
principal player in the making of the legislation known as Hatch-
Waxman. On the subject of Lewis Engman, who died in 1995, I
interviewed his wife, Pat Engman, now the head of the D.C.-
based Business Roundtable, who in turn led me to a number
of key players, all of whom were generous with their time and
thoughtful in their answers. Here I am indebted to Bob Smith and
Bob Lewis, two of Engman's closest associates; Art Amolsch,
who worked alongside Engman at the FTC; Tim Muris, the FTC
chairman in George W. Bush's first administration, who was an
Engman protégé thirty years ago; and Dr. Les Benet, who served
on a key prescription drug commission with Engman in the early
1980s. For internal FDA doings, I reviewed the entire twenty-
three-box wodge known as the "Commissioner's Chronological
Files" at the National Archives in College Park, Maryland. I
fleshed out other internal agency dynamics in interviews with
former commissioners Donald Kennedy and Jere Goyan. Dr.
Terry Kupers, now of the Wright Institute, was a key source for
medical student attitudes of the 1970s. On the subject of Henry
Waxman and his political origins, I am indebted to Francine
Kaufman, a longtime supporter of the congressman; the congressman himself also sat for a candid interview. Three invaluable sources on Hatch-Waxman were William Corr, who worked
for Waxman during the period covered; Al Engelberg, the legal genius behind generic drug litigation; and William Vodra, a former
FDA attorney and de facto historian of the period. Steve Conafay, who was Pfizer's key political operative in the 1980s, Irwin
Lerner, the former head of Roche, and Joe Williams of Parke-
Davis brilliantly described the industry side in a series of interviews. William Haddad provided a firsthand tour of his role in
the reform, via an interview and his personal papers. Romano
Romani, today a preeminent lobbyist, was generous with his
time in recounting how he and his partner, Tony Perry, prevented Senator Orrin Hatch, who did not return my calls, from
scotching the whole deal.

11   "The notion": Art Amolsch interview, February 2, 2004.

"It is not the critic who counts": Theodore Roosevelt, "Citizen-ship in a Republic" speech, Sorbonne, Paris, April 23, 1910. Bob Lewis interview, June 2003.

"The policy was never to criticize": Art Amolsch interview, Feb-ruary 2, 2004.

12   "Ralph Nader out of Adam Smith": "A Regulator to End All Reg-ulators," *Time*, July 7, 1995, p. 57.

"Much of today's regulatory machinery": Lewis A. Engman, "Consumer Is Paying Plenty," *U.S. News and World Report*, No-vember 4, 1974, p. 81.

"the consumer is paying plenty": Ibid. See also Lewis A. Eng-man, speech before the Economic Club of Detroit, Michigan, April 29, 1974.

13   "The consumer was always the bottom line": Bob Lewis inter-view, June 2003.

It was a crisis so severe as to provoke: Steve Conafay interview, April 14, 2003.

14   "What, are we supposed to schlep": Quoted in Representative Ted Weiss's "Letter to Mark Novitch, Acting FDA Commis-sioner," October 21, 1983, p. 2, in "Commissioner's Chronologi-cal Files," box 46, National Archives.

15   "In our day, it was almost an aesthetic thing": Terry Kupers in-terview, June 2003.

"At national meetings, the idea we talked about": Ibid.

"There was definitely the feeling": Steve Conafay interview, April 14, 2003.

"sat down across from me": Donald Kennedy interview, October 23, 2002.

17   "I recall him coming up to me at a fundraiser": Francine Kauf-man interview, June 2003.

"There was no way that Henry": William Corr interview, March 2003.

18   "Whenever they talked about the generics guys": Henry Wax-man interview, July 2004.

"I'll get those bastards, senator": William Haddad interview, Oc-tober 20, 2003. And see Joseph Bruce Gorman, *Kefauver: A Polit-ical Biography* (New York: Oxford University Press, 1971), pp. 298–393.

19   "It was totally immoral to insist": William Haddad interview, October 20, 2003.

"She said that not only had the numbers": Ibid.

21   "effectiveness should be found": Committee on Science and Technology, U.S. House of Representatives, "Commission on

the Federal Drug Approval Process: Final Report," 97th Cong., 2d sess., October 1982, p. 7.

21 "the FDA should provide guidance to its staff": Ibid., pp. 12–13.

"That last one was the one that really mattered": Jonah Shacknai interview, December 2, 2003.

"he could get very wound up about it": Bob Smith interview, May 14, 2003.

Bolar v. Roche: Roche Products Inc. v. Bolar Pharmaceutical Co., 733 F.2d 858 (Fed. Cir. 1984). For an outstanding account of Bolar and its political consequences, see Alfred B. Engelberg, "Special Patent Provisions for Pharmaceuticals: Have They Out-lived Their Usefulness?" *Journal of Law and Technology* (Concord, N.H.: Franklin Pierce Law Center), 1999.

22 "The companies are basically using human testing": Bob Smith interview, May 14, 2003.

"I thought Lew had gone out of his tree": Irwin Lerner interview, June 6, 2003.

"All of the sudden, these guys who had been for the deal": Bob Smith interview, May 14, 2003.

23 "generics seemed to be the right thing to do": Romano Romani interview, June 2003.

24 "He had all the tickets": Irwin Lerner interview, June 6, 2003.

"The Man in the Middle": Despite his enormous contribution to patent law and pharmaceutical industry strategy, little has been written about the career of Gerald Mossinghoff, who became the head of the PMA after the Engman affair. I interviewed him at his Alexandria offices. I then fleshed out the details of his influence in interviews with former staff, among them Bob Allnutt, and with associates such as Joe Isaacs, Myrl Weinberg, and John Peck. David Kessler, the FDA chief for much of the 1990s, refused interview requests. On the subject of the Prescription Drug User Fee Act and its impact on drug safety, Larry Sasich, the thoughtful veteran of Public Citizen, gave freely of his time. The congressional record on the hearings was detailed, pointed, and filled with outstanding primary records.

"About that, he was fresh": Joe Williams interview, May 2003.

"I remember coming to headquarters": Gerald Mossinghoff interview, April 10, 2003.

25 "a client–service provider relationship": Ibid.

"I told them, 'Look, getting new drugs approved": Ibid.

"I thought, Wow, what would it be worth": Irwin Lerner interview, June 6, 2003.

"They thought I was some kind of left-wing": Ibid.

26   "When we got to the PMA": Bob Allnutt interview, April 23, 2003.

"I recall one day getting a phone call": John Peck interview, November 25, 2003.

"A huge psychographic was blowing up": Ibid.

"our interests are synonymous with theirs": Ibid.

27   "We basically created the disease-of-the-month club": Joe Isaacs interview, November 25, 2003.

"It pushed a lot of our members": Ibid.

28   "That really helped build": Myrl Weinberg interview, May 8, 2003.

29   "We were always saying": Irwin Lerner interview, June 6, 2003.

"I said, 'Why don't we just say that the law'": Gerald Mossinghoff interview, April 10, 2003.

"For the first time, the FDA chief": Bob Allnutt interview, April 23, 2003.

30   withdrawal of its drug Omniflox: Larry Sasich interview, September 22, 2003.

"You could read between the lines": Ibid.

"has completely dried up": Ibid.

"A marketing person would tell you . . .": Ibid.

31   "a sweatshop atmosphere": Public Citizen Health Research Group, "Comments on the PDUFA," presented to the FDA, January 25, 2002, p. 1.

"It clearly follows, then, that the FDA": Committee on Energy and Commerce, House of Representatives, "Reauthorization of the Prescription Drug User Fee Act and FDA Reform," 105th Cong., 1st sess., April 23, 1997, p. 112.

"To Push the Physician's Arm": Arthur Hull Hayes, the first FDA commissioner to advocate direct-to-consumer (DTC) advertising, refused to be interviewed for this book; fortunately a number of his staff and associates did not refuse, key among them the veteran pharma legal expert Wayne Pines. The staff report by the House Committee on Energy and Commerce is a gold mine on Hayes; it contains full, unexpurgated copies of the letters pharma CEOs sent to the committee, which I quote at length. Ralph Nader's role in winning the legal right to advertise prescription drugs was detailed in a lengthy interview with Public Citizen's Alan Morrison, who argued the case in front of the Supreme Court. The story of the launch of the first DTC campaign was provided in interviews with its creator, William Castagnoli, and with Joe Davis and Jerry Weinstein. On the AMA's change of heart, I interviewed three principals, Wendy

Borow-Johnson, the head of marketing; Richard Corlin, then the chairman; and Doris Bartushka, the head of the committee charged with investigating DTC. The minutes of the meeting itself, which was attended by a number of pharmaceutical executives and FDA staff, have unfortunately been "lost," according to the AMA. On the ad industry's campaign to change the FDA's mind about DTC and off-label promotion, I conducted a series of lengthy interviews with John Kamp, arguably the architect of that campaign, and with Dan Popeo, one of the legal masterminds.

33   Hayes was instructed by the White House: Wayne Pines interview, September 29, 2003.
       It wasn't a big stretch for him: See Arthur Hull Hayes, Jr., "Remarks by Arthur Hull Hayes, Jr.," to the Pharmaceutical Advertising Council, Inc., New York, February 18, 1982.
       "among the most creative and knowledgeable people": Ibid.

34   "What patients confronted with illness want": Ibid.
       "it is my impression": Ibid.
       "we may be on the brink": Ibid.

35   "unprofessional . . . downright dangerous . . . advertising would have the objective of driving patients": All letters cited in Subcommittee on Oversight and Investigations, Committee on Energy and Commerce, House of Representatives, "Prescription Drug Advertising to Consumers: Staff Report," September 1984.
       "DTC advertising would make [patients] extraordinarily susceptible": Ibid.
       "The potential pressure of public advertising": Ibid.
       "[DTC] could adversely affect the traditional": Ibid.

36   "We believe direct advertising to the consumer": Ibid.
       "We fail to understand a benefit to *any* audience": Ibid.
       "the potential for misdirection": Ibid.
       "Would it be appropriate to push": Ibid.
       "We do not believe it is in the public health interest": Ibid.
       "dubious that the potential risks could be": Ibid.
       "consumers will come to regard": Ibid.
       "fraught with risk of consumer confusion": Ibid.

37   "battle over corporate dominance": Alan Morrison interview, September 4, 2003.
       "I realized that such a case would be more sympathetic": Ibid.

38   The core of the federal case: *Virginia State Board of Pharmacy et al. v. Virginia Citizens Consumer Council, Inc. et al.* Appeal from the United States District Court for the Eastern District of Virginia, no. 74-895. Argued November 11, 1975, decided May 24, 1976.

38   "The hearer has rights!": Alan Morrison interview, September 4, 2003.

39   "I will sell you X prescription drug at Y price": *Virginia State Board of Pharmacy.*
      "As to the particular consumer's interest in the free flow": Ibid.
      "Advertising, however tasteless and excessive": Ibid.

40   "I had understood this view to relate": Ibid.
      "Pain getting you down?": Ibid.
      "stretched my mind": Joe Davis interview, October 12, 2003.

41   "a major threat to health": Ivan Illich, *Medical Nemesis: The Expropriation of Health* (London: Marion Boyars, 1995; originally published 1975), p. 3.
      "Before sickness came to be perceived primarily as an organic": Ibid., p. 170.
      "It was one of those books that could": Joe Davis interview, October 12, 2003.

42   "They pissed all over it": William Castagnoli interview, October 17, 2003. See also, for a good history of medical advertising, William Castagnoli, *Medicine Ave.* (Huntington, N.Y.: Medical Advertising Hall of Fame, 1999).

43   "If we relied on the traditional way": Joe Davis interview, October 12, 2003.
      "Now you can put your hay fever to sleep while you stay awake!": Jerry Weinstein interview, October 2, 2003.
      "they knew everything about whiskey and cars": Joe Davis interview, October 12, 2003.

44   "They were so excited": Ibid.
      "We were idealistic": William Castagnoli interview, October 17, 2003.

45   So Cooper called an old college friend: Wendy Borow-Johnson interview, November 20, 2003.
      "a modern corporation": "James H. Sammons, M.D., Dies," *American Medical News*, July 2, 2001.
      "pointed out how inconsistent it was": Wendy Borow-Johnson interview, November 20, 2003.

46   "Times have changed": Ibid.
      "the train was leaving the station": Richard Corlin interview, March 2004. See also Proceedings of the American Medical Association, "Annual Meeting," Chicago, June 21–25, 1992.

47   Such was the case, in 1989, with the drug Tambocor: Philip J. Hilts, *Protecting America's Health: The FDA, Business, and One Hundred Years of Regulation* (New York: Alfred A. Knopf, 2003), p. 231.
      "Dr. [X]. Hello!": Sherry Danese, Regulatory Review Officer,

DDMAC, Food and Drug Administration, notice of violation letter MACMIS File #2417 to Michael J. Brennan, Associate Director, U.S. Regulatory Affairs, SmithKline, August 31, 1994.

48   "minimized adverse event data,": Sherry Danese, Regulatory Review Officer, DDMAC, FDA, Warning letter to William C. Steere, Jr., Pfizer, Inc., Chairman of the Board and CEO, August 1, 1996.

"broad spectrum efficacy": Ibid.

"promotion of unapproved uses by company sales representatives is a major problem": Mary K. Pendergast, Deputy Commissioner / Senior Advisor to the Commissioner, Statement to Subcommittee on Regulation, Business Opportunities, and Technology, Committee on Small Business, U.S. House of Representatives, October 12, 1994, p. 19.

"I asked them, 'Didn't the FDA believe'": John Kamp interview, November 24, 2003.

"We intentionally got on the speakers circuit": Ibid.

49   "government was practicing medicine": Dan Popeo interview, November 2003.

"procedures [that] are inherently chilling": *Washington Legal Foundation v. David A. Kessler and Donna Shalala*, United States District Court for the District of Columbia, July 25, 1994.

"That got Kessler's attention": John Kamp interview, November 24, 2003.

50   "Colonial Americans plainly viewed the freedom of speech": Daniel E. Troy, "History Teaches That Advertising Is More Than 'Low Value' Speech," *Commentary*, Spring 2000.

"there is no evidence . . . not be good for them": Ibid.

51   "The cases were starting to focus their minds": John Kamp interview, November 24, 2003.

"DTC advertising would make [patients] extraordinarily susceptible": Cited in Subcommittee on Oversight and Investigations, Committee on Energy and Commerce, House of Representatives, "Prescription Drug Advertising to Consumers: Staff Report," September 1984.

"Empowering the patient as well as the physician": Nancy Buc, Testimony to Department of Health and Human Services, Public Health Services, Food and Drug Administration, in "FDA Public Hearing: Direct-to-Consumer Promotion," Silver Spring, Maryland, October 18, 1995, p. 8.

52   "the ad might trigger [an] information search": Jon Schommer, Ibid., p. 2.

"I thought it was a huge mistake": Irwin Lerner interview, June 6, 2003.

52   "The brief summary is going to go the way": John Kamp inter-
      view, November 24, 2003.

53   "cannot justify a restriction of truthful, non-misleading": Guy
      Gugliotta, "FDA's Role Limited in Prescribing Drug Use," *Wash-
      ington Post*, Thursday, July 29, 1999, p. A1. See also Wayne L.
      Pines, "New Challenges for Medical Product Promotion and
      Its Regulation," *Food and Drug Law Journal*, 1997, vol. 52, pp.
      61–65.

54   "It was all supposed to be about getting": William Castagnoli in-
      terview, October 17, 2002.

55   "most medical promotion is out of sight of regulators": *Medical
      Marketing and Media*, March 2004, p. 16.
      Big Pharma Reborn: This section benefited greatly from inter-
      views with several pharmaceutical CEOs, their mentors, peers,
      and underlings. These included: SmithKline's Jan Leschly and
      his former boss at Squibb, Richard Furlaud, as well as a number
      of Leschly associates, such as Kai Lindholst and Jeremy Heyms-
      feld; Glaxo's Robert Ingram and Glaxo marketing executive John
      Dalpe; Merck's Ray Gilmartin; Lilly's Sid Taurel; Parke-Davis's
      Tony Wild and Bob Ehrlich, along with Richard Vanderveer, who
      consulted to the company's successful micromarketing program.
      Pfizer's Hank McKinnell, its current chief, refused requests for
      interviews, as did his predecessor William Steere. Fortunately
      Steere's mother, Dorothy, was helpful in constructing her son's
      early biography. An interview with Dr. Barry Bloom, Steere's
      longtime chief of research and development, outlined his boss's
      approach to that subject.

56   "The mindset was very patent-leather shoe": Bob Lewis inter-
      view, March 2003.
      "As I saw it, we had to do four things": Irwin Lerner interview,
      June 6, 2003.

57   "the end of infectious disease": For a discussion of this widely
      held postwar notion, see Richard H. Robbins, *Global Problems
      and the Culture of Capitalism* (Boston: Allyn and Bacon, 2005),
      chapter 8.
      "If you're not keeping score": Jan Leschly interview, August 31,
      1999.
      "I never stepped on the court": Ibid.

58   "Nobody danced with the other guys' wives": Kai Lindholst in-
      terview, 1996.

59   As Leschly saw it, the problem was all about perception: Jan
      Leschly interview, August 31, 1999.

60   "expanded prescribing freedom": Capoten advertisement, *New
      England Journal of Medicine*, July 3, 1986.

60   "It appears that for the first time ever a patient can feel": Ibid.
      "a job well done": Capoten advertisement, *New England Journal of Medicine*, January 21, 1988.
      "Quality of life means a feeling of well-being": Ibid.
      "means sharing love": Ibid.

61   "an extreme tolerance for mavericks": Stephen D. Moore, "Leschly Plays Offense as CEO of Kline," *Wall Street Journal*, September 7, 1994, p. B1.
      "the complete delivery of pharmaceutical care": Jan Leschly interview, Augsut 31, 1999.
      "Suddenly information technology was so essential": Ibid.

62   "I'm restructuring my work habits": David A. Garvin, "Leveraging Processes for Strategic Advantage," *Harvard Business Review*, September–October 1995, p. 88.

64   "[Brecher] said that the public press has been widely": Thomas E. Donnelly, Jr., "PAROXETINE: Suicide-Ideation and Violence-Ideation: Efficacy Review," *FDA Conversation Record*, October 3, 1990.
      "We need to set some stretch goals": Jan Leschly interview, August 31, 1999.
      "I mean, look, when I was a kid my personal goal": Ibid.

65   To pharmacologists, this meant that the drug did not act on *all*: The two best complete accounts of serotonin and supposed SSRI selectivity can be found in David Healy, *Let Them Eat Prozac: The Unhealthy Relationship between the Pharmaceutical Industry and Depression* (Toronto: James Lorimer, 2003), pp. 72–73. See also David Healy, *The Antidepressant Era* (Cambridge, Mass.: Harvard University Press, 1997).

68   "The whole world is changing!": Jan Leschly interview, August 31, 1999.
      Glaxo, the pharmaceuticals giant that ate Jan Leschly: For a brief history and timeline of Glaxo, see *http://www.gsk.com/about/background.htm*; see also Edgar Jones, *The Business of Medicine: The Extraordinary History of Glaxo, a Baby Food Producer, Which Became One of the World's Most Successful Pharmaceutical Companies* (London: Profile Books, 2001).

69   "If there is one failure it is that Tagamet exists at all": Steven Prokesch, "Glaxo's Search: Son of Zantac," *New York Times*, October 11, 1989, p. D1.

70   "would be crazy": Steve Lohr, "Glaxo Hunts a New Winner," *New York Times*, December 2, 1987, p. D1.

71   Ever since 1984, researchers studying the causes of ulcers: For a good overview of the issues, see Gina Kolata, "New Study Backs

Ulcer-Cure Theory," *New York Times*, May 6, 1992, p. C14, and David Y. Graham, "The Changing Epidemiology of GERD: Geography and *Heliobacter pylori*," *American Journal of Gastroenterology*, vol. 98, no. 7, June 2003, p. 1462.

72   "GERD is heartburn": An interview with Irwin C. Gerson conducted by William G. Castagnoli, "Looking Back. Looking Forward," *Medical Marketing and Media*, April 1998.

"GERD elevated the medical importance": Vince Parry, "The Art of Branding a Condition," *Medical Marketing and Media*, May 2003, p. 44.

"Not only did GSK double the percentage": Ibid. For examples of this kind of marketing, request a copy of *Digestive Health and Nutrition* magazine at www.dhn-online.org.

73   His ouster was likely political: Richard W. Stevenson, "In a Surprise, Glaxo's Chief Departs," *New York Times*, March 12, 1993, p. D1.

74   "These results are nothing less than staggering": Robert A. Ingram, letter to Honorable John D. Dingell in Subcommittee on Oversight and Investigations, Committee on Energy and Commerce, House of Representatives, "Prescription Drug Advertising to Consumers: Staff Report," September 1984.

"new pharmaceutical paradigm": Robert A. Ingram, "The Pharmaceutical Industry: Creating Health Instead of Treating Disease" speech, University of Mississippi's Center for Pharmaceutical Marketing and Management, State of the Industry, Jackson, Mississippi, October 6, 1998.

"creating a state of health": Ibid.

"But already today, and I believe even more so in the future": Robert Ingram interview, August 3, 1999.

"combination therapies are knocking back the viral load": Ibid.

76   But just what went on during such a session?: John Dalpe interview, August 3, 1999.

"This is a powerful sales tool": Ibid.

77   "more Relenza patients compared to placebo": Michael Elashoff, Testimony to Anti-Viral Drugs Advisory Committee Meeting, FDA, February 24, 1999.

"The fact is . . . this was an advisory committee": Robert Ingram interview, August 3, 1999.

"I was told I wouldn't be doing any more advisory committee": Michael Elashoff, *Frontline* interview, February 19, 2003.

78   new drug, Lotronex, for irritable bowel syndrome: Richard Horton, "Lotronex and the FDA: A Fatal Erosion of Integrity," *Lancet*, vol. 357, no. 9268, May 19, 2001, p. 1544.

79   In 1994, Merck, the grand old daddy: For an outstanding postwar history of the company, see Roy Vagelos and Louis Galambos, *Medicine, Science, and Merck* (Cambridge: Cambridge University Press, 2004). See also the company's own history at www.msd.com.hk/aboutus/e history of merck.html.

"showing its age": Joseph Weber, "Merck Is Showing Its Age," *Business Week*, August 23, 1993, p. 72.

80   "exhilarated": Joseph Weber, "Merck Finally Gets Its Man," *Business Week*, June 27, 1994, p. 22.

But Gilmartin did not see the complexities: Raymond Gilmartin interview, August 24, 1999. See also Raymond V. Gilmartin, "America's Healthcare Revolution: Increasing Competition and Choice, Improving People's Health" speech, Executives Club of Chicago, Chicago, Illinois, February 27, 1997; Raymond V. Gilmartin, "The Health Care Question: Global Market Solutions" speech, Economic Club of Detroit, Detroit, Michigan, March 1, 1999; Robert Berner, "Merck, CVS Join Forces on Web Site," *Wall Street Journal*, October 6, 1999.

81   "I pushed them to do extra research": Raymond Gilmartin interview, August 24, 1999.

"What matters here is how fast are you growing": Ibid.

83   "one of the fastest drug development successes in the history of Merck & Co.": Robert Zamboni, vice president medicinal chemistry, Merck, in Merck public relations release at www.merck frosst.ca/e/research/r_d/major_accomplishm/vioxx.html.

"The speed and skill with which Merck developed Vioxx": Ibid.

84   "I saw it as a new mindset": Raymond Gilmartin interview, August 24, 1999.

"health toolbox": See "MyHealth Journal," www.medcohealth.com/medco/consumer.

85   "We will always have a policy of independence for Medco": Raymond Gilmartin interview, August 24, 1999.

86   "severe": Edmund T. Pratt, Jr., "Management Report to Shareholders," 1984, p. 2.

"the company displayed a kind of promotional hoopla": "Pfizer's New Tactics for Catching Up," *Business Week*, June 16, 1973, p. 65.

87   "When Senator Kefauver attempted to grab a headline": See Samuel Mines, *Pfizer . . . An Informal History* (New York: Pfizer, 1978), pp. 208–209. For the original McKeen-Kevaufer colloquy, see "Administered Prices," Hearings before the Subcommittee on Antitrust and Monopoly, Committee on the Judiciary, United States Senate, 86th Cong., 2d sess., January 21, 22, 26, 27, 28, and 29, 1960, pp. 11216–22.

7   "women are logically emotional": Ibid.

18   "You have to pinpoint your early-adopting high writers": Sander Flaum, "Achieving a Successful Global Product Launch" speech, Pharmaceutical Marketing Congress, Philadelphia, October 2, 2002.
"You have to go to war with [FDA] for the best": Ibid.
"You have to get aggressive about creating": Ibid.
"a way to clean up your image": David Stern, "Partnering with Patient Advocacy Groups" speech, Pharmaceutical Marketing Congress, Philadelphia, October 2, 2002.

19   "third-party groups are able to make statements": Ibid.
"Increasingly, patient organizations are a way": Ibid.
"Don't hard-sell it": Ibid.
"the patient advocates are considered to be unbiased": Ibid.
"Do you know which nurse practitioners": See Blitz Research advertisement, *Medical Marketing and Media*, August 2003, p. 61.

120   "Commonhealth Confession #5": Commonhealth advertisement, *Medical Marketing and Media*, March 2004, p. 55.
Procopio, a former schoolteacher who had been attracted to health care marketing: Pat Procopio interview, September 30, 2002.
Prescriber Profiler: IMS Promotional Brochure, "IMS Marketing Effectiveness Suite: Questions. Answers. Instantly," demonstrated at Pharmaceutical Marketing Congress, Philadelphia, September 30, 2002.

122   "Brain: The World Inside Your Head": For a complete virtual tour, see www.pfizer.com/brain/etour6.html#depression.
"depression may be caused by an imbalance of neurotransmitters": Ibid.
"offers a unique platform": Braun Consulting promotional handout, Pharmaceutical Marketing Congress, Philadelphia, September 30, 2002.

123   "Sales reps enjoy full access to our mailboxes": Dan Shapiro, "Drug Companies Get Too Close for Med School's Comfort," *New York Times*, January 20, 2004, p. F5.
"a soothing oasis of the senses": "Pfizer Gives Its New Relpax Drug the Spa Treatment," *Product Marketing Today*, April 2003.

124   "the emotional space or territory a brand owns": Tom O'Dell, Grey Healthcare Group, quoted in "GHG Aims for the Heart," *Medical Marketing and Media*, September 1, 2003.
"collages depicting their feelings": Ibid.
"This is George": Ibid.

88   "There would be these very angry meetings": Steve Conafay interview, April 14, 2003.

89   "rather unfocused young man": Dorothy Steere interview, September 14, 1998.
"that he had to get on with a career . . . focused like a laser": Ibid.
"marketing had certain ideas . . . instant successes": William C. Steere, Jr., and Dr. John Niblack, "Pfizer Inc." in *Innovation: Breakthrough Ideas at 3M, DuPont, GE, Pfizer, and Rubbermaid*. Edited by Rosabeth Moss Kanter (New York: HarperBusiness, 1997), pp. 125–45.
"For the first time we, at R&D": Barry Bloom interview, November 24, 2003.

90   "Neither side was willing to yield": Steere and Niblack, *Innovation*, p. 136.

91   "He told me he had three priorities": Steve Conafay interview, April 14, 2003.
"From depression, into the mainstream": See my annotation of this slogan in Greg Critser, "Dealing a New Antidepressant," *Harper's Magazine*, May 1993, pp. 54–55.

92   "This marketing strategy produced": Healy, *Let Them Eat Prozac*, pp. 70–72.

93   "This of course made it likely that": Ibid.
"a significantly higher percentage of patients in the Rhythms group": Ibid. See also Pfizer press release archives (Pfizer.com), "Adding Education Program to Medication in Treatment of Depression Preferred by Patients," May 21, 1999.

94   "getting a little overaggressive": Cynthia Hever, of Smith Barney, quoted in Milt Freudenheim, "FDA Tells Pfizer to End Claims," *New York Times*, August 8, 1996, p. D1.
"immediately cease": Sherry Danese, Regulatory Review Officer, DDMAC, Food and Drug Administration, Warning letter to William C. Steere, Jr., Pfizer, Inc., August 1, 1996.
"within 15 days of the date of this letter, disseminate": Ibid.
"We already have many ways of drilling down to patients": William Steere, quoted in *Pharmaceutical Executive*, October 1995, p. 3; and cited in Greg Critser, "Oh, How Happy We Will Be," *Harper's Magazine*, June 1996, pp. 39–48.

95   "Viagra crystallized some things I'd been thinking": David Stipp, "Why Pfizer Is So Hot," *Fortune*, May 11, 1998.

96   "Be pioneering!": Richard Vanderveer interview, September 19, 2003.
"a serious problem": Milt Freudenheim, "Warner-Lambert Falls after Vote by Panel," *New York Times*, October 19, 1988, p. D4.

97 "I told Joe that he needed to institute a micromarketing": Richard Vanderveer interview, September 19, 2003.

98 "put the detail person in a simpatico headset with the doctor": Ibid.

"He was a happy executive": Ibid. See also Richard B. Vanderveer, "The Shameful State of Pharmaceutical Marketing," *Medical Marketing and Media*, September 1, 1995.

100 "The low-risk approach can end up as the high-risk approach": Anthony Wild interview, November 16, 2003.

"the sales force is too small": Ibid.

"We decided to hold a national sales conference": Ibid.

"Why are all these caps here?": Ibid.

'Why?' Why not let them get rich?": Ibid.

101 "We announced we were taking off": Ibid.

102 "At Parke-Davis, many of the medical liaisons": Dr. David Franklin, "Affidavit of David Franklin," in *United States of America ex rel. David Franklin v. Pfizer, Inc., and Parke-Davis, Division of Warner-Lambert Company*, Civil Action No. 96-11651-PBS, p. 2.

103 "if you get caught violating the FDA": "Disclosure of Information by Relator David P. Franklin," Ibid., pp. 7–9.

"We expect you to do your job out there": Ibid.

"The only way we will make it [to the Bahamas]": Ibid.

105 "I want you out there every day selling Neurontin": Ibid., p. 11.

107 "we had a very clever regulatory crew": Anthony Wild interview, November 16, 2003.

"When I arrived, the sales forecast for Lipitor": Ibid.

108 "from gum to Tums": Robert Ehrlich interview, October 8, 2003.

"We had a fairly good efficacy advantage": Ibid.

"Instead, we took a consumer insight": Ibid.

109 "There was a missing discussion": Ibid.

"To the consumer, it was 'I can reduce my shots'": Ibid.

"brazen criminal behavior": "Disclosure of Information by Relator David P. Franklin," p. 8.

2. We Love It!

The task of getting inside pharmaceutical marketing was greatly aided by attendance at several pharma and medical conferences and congresses. Among them were the annual Pharmaceutical Marketing Congress, held in Philadelphia in 2002; the annual Pharmaceutical Research and Development Summit, held in Phoenix in 2004; the 2003 convention of the American Psychiat-

ric Association, this one held in San Francisco; convention of the American Society of Clinical and Therapeutics, held in Washington, D.C., in 20 dustry trade magazines have been helpful as well, *Product Marketing Today* to *Medical Marketing Pharmaceutical Executive*.

111 "I was wrong about DTC": "News from the D Conference and Exposition," *DTC Perspectives*, Ma p. 10.

Citing a study by the Kaiser Family Foundation: Ibi

112 "the most serious conditions": Ibid.

The industry group Rx Insight: Ibid.

113 Heads of marketing from traditional consumer goods 25 Marketers," *DTC Perspectives*, May–June 2002, p

"Our markets, customers, and products are all unde Patrick Kelly, Keynote speech, to Pharmaceutical Congress, Philadelphia, September 30, 2002.

114 "It's time to fight back!": Ibid.

"We are challenged that our products": Ibid.

"in that way we can move toward the spiritual-ethical Ibid.

"We must find a way to market beyond just product": I

"We have to figure out the modern patient's real needs'

115 "There are still a profound number of patients who don Ibid.

"We have to use that to push them into the camp": Ibid.

116 "All great drugs create tribes!": Patrick Dixon's slid "Looking Towards the Future of the Pharmaceutical In www.globalchange.com/cv.htm.

"If you do a hundred sixty days of DTC ads": Raymond Sa "Patient Compliance and Adherence Marketing" speech maceutical Marketing Congress, Philadelphia, Septem 2002.

117 "The doctor sits *in loco parentis*": Ibid.

"physician who does not feel comfortable with a drug" Roberts, "Using Multi-Channel CRM Strategies," panel sion at Pharmaceutical Marketing Congress, Philadelphia tember 30, 2002.

"Traditionally, women are seekers": Gail Ludmeyer, "Mark to Women: The Cutting Edge of Pharmaceutical Market panel discussion at Pharmaceutical Marketing Congress, P delphia, September 30, 2002.

125   Effexor XR: "Silver Winner," *Product Management Today*, October 2003, p. 19.

       "AstraZeneca actually had to teach the market": Ibid.

126   "Nearly 80 percent of all clinical studies": Frank Kilpatrick, "Rev Up Patient Recruitment," *Pharmaceutical Executive*, April 1, 2002.

127   "A multifunctional team should be established": Bruce Shutan, "Getting Marketing Mileage from Clinical Trials," *Product Management Today*, October 2003, p. 30.

       "Marketing and commercial development work together": Ibid., p. 31.

       "Gone are the days when companies just handed": "PR Power," *Pharmaceutical Executive*, September 2002, p. 9.

129   "A Radical Proposal": Frank S. Kilpatrick and Malcolm Bohm, "A New Clinical Trial Process Interaction Model" presentation, R&D Drug Development Summit, Phoenix, February 9, 2004.

       "We have to understand — really get wet in the field": Ibid.

       "mentors . . . in nonalignment": Ibid.

130   "Academic entities might not provide": Ibid.

       "deploying clinical fieldworkers to locate marginalized patients": Ibid. See also Kilpatrick, "Rev Up Patient Recruitment."

131   "At an approximate cost of $600,000": Ibid. Also presentation by Frank Kilpatrick and Malcolm Bohm, February 9, 2004.

       "One, the money": Alison MacPherson interview, May 9, 2004.

       "One third of clinical trial volunteers": "Will Physicians Refer Their Patients into Clinical Trials?," *CenterWatch Monthly*, vol. 11, no. 3, March 2004, p. 1.

132   "Are you a single gorgeous woman": Advertisement in *LA Weekly*, September 5–11, 2003, p. 54.

134   *New Life Live*: Listen for yourself at www.newlifelive.com.

136   "humanity's depravity": Ibid. See also Frank Minirth and Paul Meier, *Happiness Is a Choice: The Symptoms, Causes, and Cures of Depression* (Grand Rapids, Mich.: Baker Books, 2d ed., 1994); Paul Meier, Stephen Arterburn, and Frank Minirth, *Mood Swings: Understand Your Emotional Highs and Lows and Achieve a More Balanced and Fulfilled Life* (Nashville: Thomas Nelson, 1999).

       "Psychiatry and Christianity have never experienced better superficial": Dan Blazer, *Freud vs. God: How Psychiatry Lost Its Soul and Christianity Lost Its Mind* (Downers Grove, Ill., InterVarsity Press, 1998), p. 13.

137   "The media's increased coverage of health topics": Keith J. Petrie, "Modern Worries, New Technology, and Medicine," *Brit-*

ish Medical Journal, vol. 324, March 23, 2002, pp. 690–91. See also Keith J. Petrie et al., "Thoroughly Modern Worries: The Relationship of Worries About Modernity to Reported Symptoms, Health and Medical Care Utilization," *Journal of Psychosomatic Research,* vol. 51, July 2001, pp. 395–401.

137 "People now feel much more vulnerable": Petrie, "Thoroughly Modern Worries," p. 690.

139 "All forms of organizational instability, including rapid expansion": Hugo Westerlund et al., "Workplace Expansion, Long-Term Sickness Absence, and Hospital Admission," *Lancet,* vol. 363, April 10, 2004, p. 1193.

"Repeated exposure to rapid personnel expansion": Ibid. See also Hugo Westerlund et al., "Organizational Instability and Cardiovascular Risk Factors in White-Collar Employees," *European Journal of Public Health,* March 14, 2004; "Why Business Is Bad for Your Health," editorial in *Lancet,* vol. 363, April 10, 2004. On the connection between job stress and hypertension, see P. L. Schnall et al., "The Relationship Between 'Job Strain,' Workplace Diastolic Blood Pressure, and Left Ventricular Mass Index," *JAMA,* vol. 263, no. 14, April 11, 1990, pp. 1929–35.

"higher turnover, more individual (as opposed to collective) demands": Westerlund, "Workplace Expansion," p. 1197.

140 The short history: For this information I have relied heavily on the work of Lawrence H. Diller, M.D., and his well-rounded *Running on Ritalin* (New York, Bantam Books, 1998). For a pointed argument against Ritalin, see Richard DeGrandpre, *Ritalin Nation* (New York: W. W. Norton, 2000). For the sociology of Ritalin, see Neil Howe and William Strauss, *Millennials Rising: The Next Great Generation* (New York: Vintage Books, 2000).

141 "It was not amphetamine": Diller, *Running on Ritalin,* p. 25.

142 Between 1989 and 1991, sales fell by 37 percent: Ibid., p. 42.

143 "the single biggest factor in the explosion of ADD diagnosis": Ibid., p. 315.

145 Spending on all forms of drugs to treat childhood and adolescent: Milt Freudenheim, "Behavior Drugs Lead in Sales for Children," *New York Times,* May 17, 2004, p. C9.

146 "She's not refilling her prescriptions": RTC Relationship Marketing advertisement, *DTC Perspectives,* May–June 2002, p. 55.

"Bennington tends to be more bulimic": Gertrude Carter interview, March 3, 2004.

"The percent of students seeking help": Ibid.

147 "Those records are typically horrendous": Ibid.

"These fractured interactions with caregivers": Gertrude Carter and Jeffrey Winseman, "The Illusion of Certainty: Do Advances in Psychopharmacology Suggest That Students' Inner Lives Are Irrelevant?" *Chronicle of Higher Education*, August 3, 2001, p. B2.

147 "Kaiser Permanente, one of the first HMOs": Ibid.

148 "not to promote Ritalin": Gertrude Carter interview, March 3, 2004.

"Students who request medicine for their problems": Carter and Winseman, "The Illusion of Certainty," p. B2.

"There are more young people who can succeed": Ed Weismeier interview, January 22, 2004.

"the old relationship of mutual communication": Gary Margolis interview, February 25, 2004.

149 "the California cocktail": Norman Hoffman interview, March 10, 2004.

150 "back in 1993, [counseling centers] were still running": Richard Keeling interview, March 10, 2004.

"Development of School-based Adolescent Depression Awareness Program": Karen L. Schwartz et al., American Psychiatric Association annual meeting, San Francisco, May 20, 2003.

151 "We are entering what could be the golden age": Quoted in Robert Steinbrook, "Testing Medications in Children," *New England Journal of Medicine*, vol. 347, no. 18, October 31, 2002, p. 1462.

153 "What do D's in school, increased risk of driving accidents": Kathryn Mayurnik, "What Do D's . . ." media alert, Fleishman-Hillard Agency, May 20, 2003.

"Continuous symptom relief is the key message": David Shaffer, Eli Lilly, speech to APA, May 20, 2003.

"outlining your map to productivity": Robert Tudisco, "Focus on Adults with ADHD," *Attention!*, February 2003, p. 10.

154 "ADHD is not a disease, it's an organizational disorder": Calvin Sumner interview, May 20, 2003.

"Of particular interest to researchers": Matt McMillen, "Paying Attention to Adult ADHD," *Attention!* February 2003, p. 27. For an outstanding overview of ADHD in the workplace, see Lisa Belkin, "Office Messes," *New York Times Magazine*, July 18, 2004, p. 24.

155 "Half of all office workers sleep poorly": Arlene Weintraub, "I Can't Sleep," *Business Week*, January 26, 2004, p. 66.

156 "In terms of error rate, 18 hours of no sleep": Anahad O'Connor, "Wakefulness Finds a Powerful Ally," *New York Times*, June 29, 2004, p. D1.

157 "lying down to rest in the afternoon": Cephalon Inc., "The Epworth Sleepiness Scale (ESS)" at www.provigil.com.

157   "No one would ever have believed it would be this big": O'Connor, "Wakefulness Finds a Powerful Ally," p. D3.

158   "The drug enables us to be that much more workaholic": Ibid, p. D1.
      "The natural checks on that tendency": Ibid.

159   "fifth vital sign": This is the official tagline of the American Pain Society.
      first-time abusers of opioids: Office of Applied Studies, SAMHSA, Drug Abuse Warning Network, "The Dawn Report: Oxycodone, Hydrocodone, and Polydrug Use, 2002," July 2004.

160   "What we are seeing now are bright": Dr. Clifford Bernstein interview, September 15, 2000.
      "All of the attributes of the winner": David Crausman interview, September 16, 2000. See also Greg Critser, "Pill Shaves Off Life's Edges — at a Price," USA Today, October 2, 2000, p. 19A.

161   In taverns, Glaxo circulated coasters and glasses: Nat Ives, "A Different Tack on Heartburn: Go on, Indulge," New York Times, June 10, 2004, p. C1.

162   In long-term-care homes: Jake Levine and Therese Zanglin, "Long-Term Care Market Growth and the Drug Industry Response," Product Management Today, May 2003, pp. 20–21.

164   "It is not a sufficiently accurate predictor": Ray Moynihan et al., "Selling Sickness: The Pharmaceutical Industry and Disease Mongering," British Medical Journal, vol. 324, April 13, 2002, p. 889.

165   "I cannot agree with that at all": Sidney Taurel interview, August 15, 1999.
      "Today, less than nineteen percent of Americans over sixty-five": Sidney Taurel, "The Future of Aging: Social Consequences of the Biomedical Revolution" speech, Town Hall, Los Angeles, March 2, 2004.

166   "Retirees today are not buying rocking chairs": Ibid.
      "Basically, we are building new bone": Sidney Taurel interview, March 2, 2004.
      Such was the approach of Dr. Bob Arnot's: Dr. Bob Arnot, The Breast Cancer Prevention Diet: The Powerful Foods, Supplements, and Drugs That Can Save Your Life (Boston: Little, Brown, 1998).
      "mental exercise": William Rodman Shankle, M.S., M.D., and Daniel G. Amen, M.D., Preventing Alzheimer's: Ways to Help Prevent, Delay, Detect, and Even Halt Alzheimer's Disease and Other Forms of Memory Loss (New York: G. P. Putnam's Sons, 2004), p. 145.

167   "Staying young is the new American dream": Steven Lamm,

M.D., and Gerald Secor Couzens, *Younger at Last: Discover the Age-Defying Powers of Vitality Medicine* (New York: Pocket Books, 1997), p. 1.

167   "In your search, you are going to come across physicians": Ibid., p. 3.

"fast-acting with virtually no side effects": Steven Lamm, M.D., and Gerald Secor Couzens, *The Virility Solution: Everything You Need to Know About the FDA-Approved Potency Pill That Can Restore and Enhance Male Sexuality* (New York: Simon and Schuster, 1998), p. 70.

168   neoclassical spa that resembles the White House: Andrea Petersen, "Finding a Cure for Old Age," *Wall Street Journal*, May 20, 2003, p. D8.

3. The Full Price

A number of texts on the subject of drug-induced injury informed this section, none more so than Neil Kaplowitz and Laurie D. Deleve's definitive *Drug-Induced Liver Disease*. The principal medical journals were also of great help, among them the *Journal of the American Medical Association*, *Archives of Internal Medicine*, *The Lancet*, *The New England Journal of Medicine*, *Pediatrics*, *The Cleveland Clinic Journal of Medicine*, *Clinical Pharmacology and Therapeutics*, *The British Medical Journal*, and *Archives of General Psychiatry*. Dr. Jay S. Cohen's outstanding but overlooked book, *Over Dose: The Case Against the Drug Companies* (New York: Tarcher-Putnam, 2001), was also helpful. The definitive *Principles of Clinical Pharmacology*, edited by Dr. Arthur Atkinson and others, aided in my understanding of clinical pharmacology. I interviewed Dr. Atkinson, as well as Dr. Barbara Levey, at the time the president of the American Society of Clinical Pharmacology and Therapeutics. My interviews with the FDA's Dr. David Graham, with Vanderbilt University's Alastair Wood, and with Dr. Jonathan Wright on the subject of drug safety were helpful, as were conversations with Lilly's Dr. Steve Paul and Dr. Andrew Dahlem. The agency provided transcripts of hearings. I drew all court testimony from original court documents.

171   "the end of the sanguine empire": Thomas Bartholin, *Lymphatic Vessels*, 1653, quoted in Stanford University's "History of the Body" Web site, www.Stanford.edu/class/history13/early sciencelab/body/liver pages.

liver primer: An outstanding layman's primer can be found in

Howard J. Worman, *The Liver Disorders Sourcebook* (Los Angeles: Lowell House, 1999).

173   "People are taking more and more drugs": John R. Senior interview, April 3, 2003.

"In the United States drug-induced liver disease": Neil Kaplowitz, "Drug-Induced Liver Disorders: Introduction and Overview," *Drug-Induced Liver Disease*, ed. by Neil Kaplowitz and Laurie D. Deleve (New York, Marcel Dekker, 2003), pp. 1, 8, and 9.

"To identify acute liver failure": Ibid., p. 9.

174   "very emotional": Concepción Morgado, testimony in *Concepción Morgado v. Warner-Lambert Co., Parke-Davis and Co., and Pfizer, Inc.*, March 11, 2003, U.S. District Court, Southern District Court of New York (MDL-1348).

175   "Your breath, it's really . . . *bad*": Lazarro Morgado, Ibid.

"Your blood sugar is totally uncontrolled": Dr. Jaime Lara, Ibid.

"You're going back on the drugs": Ibid.

"Will increase to 4 milligrams, then try Rezulin?": Ibid.

176   open-door policy at the FDA: See David Willman's Pulitzer Prize–winning series in the *Los Angeles Times*, "Rezulin: Hidden Risks, Lethal Truths," June 30, 2002, p. A1.

"a pile of shit": Mary E. Taylor, testimony in *Gerald Marza v. Warner-Lambert*, Galveston County, Texas, May 21, 2002.

177   "I mean I had experience with medications": Dr. Jaime Lara, *Morgado v. Warner-Lambert*.

178   "easy for them to take the high road": Anthony Wild letter quoted in Willman, "Rezulin: Hidden Risks, Lethal Truths," p. A1.

"When I got up, all the energy flew down": Concepción Morgado, *Morgado v. Warner-Lambert*.

179   "Number one is the fatigues that she has": Dr. Jaime Lara, Ibid.

180   "She doesn't wait for me today": Lazarro Morgado, Ibid.

"intentionally and recklessly misrepresent[ed]": Jury finding, Ibid.

"Warner-Lambert act[ed] wantonly and recklessly": Ibid.

"All the . . . signal[s] were present": Kaplowitz, "Drug-Induced Liver Disorders," p. 9.

181   "He liked to tell people that he still quoted a Zimmerman": Rochelle Sharpe, "How a Drug Approved by the FDA Turned into Lethal Failure," *Wall Street Journal*, Sept 30, 1998, p. A1. See also William M. Lee, "Drug-Induced Hepatotoxicity," *New England Journal of Medicine*, vol. 349, no. 5, July 31, 2003, p. 483.

183   "The levels of risk exceed those of Rezulin": David Graham interview, September 22, 2003.

184   "We could not understand why David": Larry Sasich interview,
        September 22, 2003.
        "Everyone [at the Arava safety committee meeting] came from
        a reviewing background": David Graham interview, September
        22, 2003.
        "They get subjected to an incredible amount of pressure": Ibid.

185   "Dosing is the single most important": Alastair Wood interview,
        July 24, 2002.
        "The drug companies are scared to death of it": Ibid. See also
        Nancy J. Olsen et al., "New Drugs for Rheumatoid Arthritis,"
        New England Journal of Medicine, vol. 350, no. 21, May 20,
        2004, p. 2169.

187   The diet drug Redux was a grim case: For this summary, I have
        relied on the work of Alicia Mundy, Dispensing with the Truth:
        The Victims, the Drug Companies, and the Dramatic Story Be-
        hind the Battle over Fen-Phen (New York: St. Martin's Press,
        2001).

190   "The potential advantage of decreasing the risk": Review of FDA
        Center for Drug Evaluation Research (CDER) Arthritis Advisory
        Committee Meeting, "Celebrex and Vioxx," February 7–8, 2001.
        "The Alleged Benefits of Celecoxib and Rofecoxib: A Scientific
        Fraud": Xavier Bosch, "Spanish Editor Sued over Rofecoxib Alle-
        gations," Lancet, vol. 363, no. 9414, January 24, 2004, p. 298.
        "accurately reflects the reports of serious methodological": Judg-
        ment, Madrid Court of First Instance, Oral Hearing 965/2002,
        January 22, 2004.

191   "was associated with an unanticipated fivefold": Cited in Eric J.
        Topol and Gary W. Falk, "A Coxib a Day Won't Keep the Doctor
        Away," Lancet, vol. 364, no. 9435, August 21, 2004, pp. 639–40.
        For a succinct, illustrated explanation of one way COX-2 drugs
        cause blood clots, see Aaron J. Marcus et al., "COX Inhibitors
        and Thromboregulation," New England Journal of Medicine,
        vol. 347, no. 13, September 26, 2002, pp. 1025–26.
        "The coxib field had been marked by intensive DTC advertis-
        ing": Ibid.

193   The NIH, backed by the top heart-related medical organizations:
        Gina Kolata, "Experts Set a Lower Low for Cholesterol Levels,"
        New York Times, July 13, 2004, p. A1. See also Antonio M.
        Gotto, "Safety and Statin Therapy," Archives of Internal Medi-
        cine, vol. 163, March 24, 2003, pp. 657–59, and Paul Thompson
        et al., "Statin-Associated Myopathy," JAMA, vol. 289, no. 13,
        April 2, 2003, pp. 1681–90.

194   Yet it is at higher doses of statins that problems": James A. de
        Lemos et al., "Early Intensive Versus Delayed Conservative

Simvastatin Strategy in Patients with Acute Coronary Syndromes," *JAMA*, vol. 292, no. 11, September 15, 2004, p. 292.

195 The ACE inhibitors fared most poorly: ALLHAT officers and co-ordinators for the ALLHAT Collaborative Research Group, "Major Outcomes in High-Risk Hypertensive Patients Randomized to Anglotensin-Converting Enzyme Inhibitor or Calcium Channel Blocker vs. Diuretic. The Antihypertensive and Lipid-Lowering Treatment to Prevent Heart Attack Trial (ALLHAT)," *JAMA*, vol. 288, no. 23, 2002, pp. 2981–97.

96 percent of authors in favor: Henry Thomas Stelfox et al., "Conflict of Interest in the Debate Over Calcium-Channel Antagonists," *New England Journal of Medicine*, vol. 338, no. 2, January 8, 1998, pp. 101–6. Cited in Melody Petersen, "Diuretics' Value Drowned Out by Trumpeting of Newer Drugs," *New York Times*, December 18, 2002, p. A32.

196 Somewhere between 3 and 20 percent: Metin Ozkan et al., "Drug-Induced Lung Disease," *Cleveland Clinic Journal of Medicine*, vol. 68, no. 9, September 2001, pp. 782–91.

197 In January 2004, the Japanese Ministry of Health: "Arthritis Drug Tied to Five Deaths," *Japan Times*, January 28, 2004 (www.japantimes.com).

Worldwide, there have now been eighty cases: Justin McCurry, "Japan Deaths Spark Concerns Over Arthritis Drug," *Lancet*, vol. 363, no. 9407, February 7, 2004, p. 461.

199 too *little* stomach acid can be just as bad: Jonathan V. Wright and Lane Lenard, *Why Stomach Acid Is Good for You* (New York: M. Evans, 2001).

"It was revealing in so many ways": Jonathan V. Wright interview, November 25, 2003.

200 Of the Prilosec patients who had *H. pylori*: Wright and Lenard, *Why Stomach Acid Is Good for You*, pp. 92, 93.

"In principal, current [acid-suppressing drug] therapies": Ibid., p. 93.

201 "People will end up with diseases in their sixties": Jonathan V. Wright interview, November 25, 2003.

In October 2004, two of the nation's leading gastroenterologists: Robert J. F. Laheij, "Risk of Community-Acquired Pneumonia and Use of Gastric-Acid Suppressive Drugs," *New England Journal of Medicine*, vol. 292, no. 16, October 27, 2004, pp. 1955–60.

202 "More than 70 percent of all *Physicians' Desk Reference* entries": Jeffrey L. Blumer, "Off-Label Uses of Drugs in Children," *Pediatrics*, vol. 104, no. 3, September 1999, p. 598.

"We were advised with great authority that Matt was suffering": Mark Miller, testimony to Food and Drug Administration Advisory Panel on Antidepressants and Pediatric Use, February 2, 2004, p. 341.

203 "The internist who saw him for thirty minutes prescribed Paxil": Alice Erber in Ibid., p. 365.

204 "This was a young woman who had everything to live for": Sara Bostock in Ibid., p. 294.

"no suicidal ideation": Gary Cheslek in Ibid., February 2, 2004, p. 143.

"He didn't leave a note": Ibid.

"some people will never get enough information": Jan Leschly interview, August 31, 1999.

206 "There have been 677 trials involving SSRIs": David Healy, testimony to Food and Drug Administration Advisory Panel on Antidepressants and Pediatric Use, February 2, 2004, p. 383.

"They were only doing what Lilly and Pfizer had already done": Ibid.

207 Any foreign substance that interacts with such malleable cerebral structures: Kimberly Goldapple et al., "Modulation of Cortical-Limbic Pathways in Major Depression," *Archives of General Psychiatry*, vol. 61, no. 1, 2004, pp. 34–41. See also Gregory L. Kearns et al., "Developmental Pharmacology — Drug Disposition, Action, and Therapy in Infants and Children," *New England Journal of Medicine*, vol. 349, no. 12, September 18, 2003, pp. 1157–67, and Jeffrey L. Blumer, "Off-Label Uses of Drugs in Children," *Pediatrics*, vol. 104, no. 3, September 1999, pp. 598–602.

"The problem is that our usage has outstripped our knowledge": Jeffrey Kluger, "Medicating Young Minds," *Time*, November 3, 2003, p. 58.

208 Between 1997, when the law was passed, and 2001: Cited in Alice Dembner, "Dangerous Dosage," *Boston Globe*, February 18, 2001, p. A1. See also Mark Mathieu, *New Drug Approval in the United States* (Waltham, Mass.: Parexel, 2002), pp. 319–45.

209 "They told me they were just trying to see how effective": Dembner, "Dangerous Dosage."

210 "significant inflammation": Ibid.

211 "sounded happy": J. K. Wall and John Toohy, "Woman Participating in Lilly Trial Hangs Self," *Indianapolis Star*, February 9, 2004, p. A1.

potent inhibitor of cytochrome P450: For a discussion of Cymbalta and cytochrome P4502D6, see Michael H. Skinner et al., "Duloxetine Is Both an Inhibitor and a Substrate of Cytochrome P4502D6 in Healthy Volunteers," *Clinical Pharmacology and Therapeutics*, vol. 73, no. 3, March 2003, p. 170.

212 "I think you are saying, 'Should we be careful'": Steve Paul interview, March 2, 2004.

213 In 2004, researchers from the NIH performed an intricate: R. J. Edison and M. Muenke, "Central Nervous System and Limb Anomalies in Case Reports of First Trimester Statin Exposure," *New England Journal of Medicine*, vol. 350, no. 15, April 8, 2004, pp. 1579–82.

"The unfortunate reality is that we learn about virtually": Allen A. Mitchell, "Systematic Identification of Drugs That Cause Birth Defects — A New Opportunity," *New England Journal of Medicine*, vol. 349, no. 26, December 25, 2003, p. 2556.

"Operating without overarching guidance": Ibid.

216 percentage of elderly patients receiving *nine or more*: Cited in Jim Rosack, "Catastrophic Medication Interactions Plague Elderly, Demand Solutions," *Psychiatric News*, October 20, 2000, p. 1.

"Most individuals who are prescribed five or more drugs": Steven F. Werder, "Managing Polypharmacy: Walking the Fine Line Between Help and Harm," *Current Psychiatry*, vol. 2, no. 2, February 2003, p. 1.

"A medication — drug number 1 — causes an adverse effect": Cited in Rosack, "Catastrophic Medication Interactions," p. 2.

217 "significant anticholinergic activity": Jacobo Mintzer and Alistair Burns, "Anticholinergic Side Effects of Drugs in Elderly People," *Journal of the Royal Society of Medicine*, vol. 93, September 2000, pp. 457–62.

"reversible confusional states": Ibid., p. 458.

"In practice, the information available": Ibid., p. 460.

"cholinergic bomb": *Psychiatric News*, October 20, 2000 (www.psych.org/pnews).

218 "are known to cause harm or induce harmful side effects": Lesley Curtis et al., "Inappropriate Prescribing for Elderly Americans in a Large Outpatient Population," *Archives of Internal Medicine*, vol. 164, no. 15, August 9/23, 2004, pp. 1621–25.

"known to cause drug-drug interactions": David N. Juurlink et al., "Drug-Drug Interactions Among Elderly Patients Hospitalized for Drug Toxicity," *JAMA*, vol. 289, no. 13, April 2, 2003, p. 1652.

"More than 40 percent of all benzodiazepines": Olivera J. Boqunovic, M.D., and Shelly F. Greenfield, M.D., M.P.H., "Practical Geriatrics: Use of Benzodiazepines Among the Elderly," *Journal of the American Psychiatric Association*, March 2004, p. 283.

219 "Perhaps because most physicians in practice today had little":

Knight Steel, "Comment," *Archives of Internal Medicine*, vol. 164, no. 15, August 9/23, 2004.

219   "Is there too great a willingness": Ibid.

4. The End of the Great Buffer?

The subject of physicians and drug company influence has slowly begun to inspire popular writing by medical authorities. A valuable, opinionated volume is longtime *New England Journal of Medicine* editor Marcia Angell's *The Truth About the Drug Companies* (Random House, 2004). Another is Jerry Avorn's *Powerful Medicines: The Benefits, Risks, and Costs of Prescription Drugs* (Knopf, 2004). On the subject of lobbying, this section benefited from the wisdom of two key industry players, the former Pfizer political chief Steve Conafay and the former PhRMA medical affairs adviser Bert Spilker. William Vodra, a longtime industry attorney and thoughtful observer, now at Arnold and Porter, gave me a real-world look at how regulatory politics operates in modern Washington, as did Peter Barton Hutt, also a former FDA attorney who has long occupied the upper realm of pharma legaldom. I based my discussion of Dan Troy on interviews with associates and on FDA documents obtained via the Freedom of Information Act. Troy refused to be interviewed. And my discussion of the industry's self-inflicted wounds benefited enormously from attendance, in 2003, of the Financial Times Global Pharmaceutical Conference; I quote and summarize the speeches and comments of several CEOs and senior executives there.

221   A recently published account by a former Viagra: Jamie Reidy, *Hard Sell* (Kansas City: Andrews McMeel, 2005), p. 173.
      "7:45 A.M. — Attend grand rounds at the hospital": Lisa Lane, *3 Days to a Pharmaceutical Sales Job Interview*, 3d. edition (Clarksburg, N.J.: Lisa Lane and Drug Careers, 2003), p. 80.

222   why some 90 percent of all CME classes: David Blumenthal, "Doctors and Drug Companies," *New England Journal of Medicine*, vol. 351, no. 18, October 28, 2004, pp. 1885–90.

223   "when suddenly they see the patient as an equal": Louis Lasagna, *Life, Death and the Doctor* (New York: Alfred A. Knopf, 1968), p. 252.
      "Feelings of obligation are not related to the size": Blumenthal, "Doctors and Drug Companies," p. 1887.
      "have trouble seeing themselves as biased": Ibid.
      marketing executives at Schering-Plough: Gardiner Harris, "As

Doctor Writes Prescription, Drug Company Writes a Check,"
New York Times, Sunday, June 27, 2004, p. A1.

224 "the resulting changes in the use of medication": Blumenthal,
p. 1880.

"Interestingly . . . the larger the number of gifts": Ibid., p. 1888.

225 "persuasion, kind, unassuming persuasion": Jim Barnett, "The
Monday Profile: Alan Holmer," *Oregonian*, October 18, 2004,
p. A1.

"We must keep our lines of communication open": Sheryl Gay
Stolberg and Gardiner Harris, "Industry Fights to Put Imprint on
Drug Bill," *New York Times*, September 5, 2003, p. A1.

"donate the maximum": Ibid.

226 "changing the Canadian health care system": Robert Pear, "Drug
Companies Increase Spending on Efforts to Lobby Congress and
Governments," *New York Times*, June 1, 2003, p. A33.

"Can you believe that?": Steve Conafay interview, June 2, 2003.

228 "When I got the list back from circulation": Bert Spilker interview, July 26, 2002.

"I had a strong sense that, if the president signs on": Alastair
Wood interview, July 24, 2002.

"One of the lessons that came out of this for me": Ibid.

229 "We shouldn't be averse to risk": Dr. Lester Crawford interview,
August 6, 2002. See also "The JIM Interview: Lester Crawford,
Jr., D.V.M., Ph.D.," *Journal of Investigative Medicine*, vol. 50,
no. 4, July 2002, pp. 247–49, and "We Shouldn't Be Risk Averse,"
PharmaTimes, July/August 2002.

"The industry would be pleased if Les would become": Bert
Spilker interview, July 26, 2002.

"posed no excess health risks for patients": Abigail Zuger, "Rx:
Canadian Drugs," *New England Journal of Medicine*, vol. 349,
no. 23, December 4, 2003, pp. 2188–90.

230 "We won't bite": Warren R. Ross, "Mark McClellan and Peter
Pitts, the Top Officials of the FDA, Would Like the Adversarial
Relationship with the Pharma Industry to End. But Just How
Friendly Can Regulators Be?" *Medical Marketing and Media*,
January 2004, p. 20.

"how to push the promotional envelope": Ibid., p. 22.

in 2003 DDMAC issued drug makers 75 percent fewer: "U.S.
FDA Sends Fewer Warnings on Drug Ads," Reuters, October 1,
2003.

"Most Medical Promotion Is Out of Sight of Regulators": Troy
had made more than $350,000: Daniel Troy, "Schedule D, 2001:
Executive Branch Personnel Public Financial Disclosure Re

port," June 30, 2003 (document obtained through Freedom of Information Act).

231   "can harm public health": See in re. Paxil Litigation, 01-07937, and see in re. *Motus v. Pfizer, Inc.* 02-55372, September 2002. For a summary, see also Robert Pear, "In a Shift, Bush Moves to Block Medical Suits," *New York Times*, Sunday, July 25, 2004, p. A1.

233   "The contributions of pharmaceutical manufacturers that provide financial assistance": John K. Iglehart, "The New Medicare Prescription-Drug Benefit — A Pure Power Play," *New England Journal of Medicine*, vol. 350, no. 8, February 19, 2004, pp. 826–33.

234   "I'm certainly not the person to determine whether Paxil": Gardiner Harris, "Spitzer Sues a Drug Maker, Saying It Hid Negative Data," *New York Times*, June 3, 2004, p. A1.

235   The whistleblower tactic is now being imitated around the country: Alex Berenson, "Trial Lawyers Are Now Focusing on Lawsuits Against Drug Makers," *New York Times*, Sunday, May 18, 2003, p. A1.
        huge confabs of them gathered in giant meeting places: Ibid.

236   "You would think that a party with their wives": Gardiner Harris, "Fractured Image in Need of Mending for Drug Makers," *New York Times*, July 8, 2004, p. C1.
        "This industry delivered miracles": Ibid. For an example of a company trying to change its ability to discover drugs, see Richard C. Morais, "Mind the Gap," *Forbes*, August 11, 2003, p. 58. For a discussion of new drug discovery rates, see "Is Science Stuck in the Middle Ages?" *Lancet*, vol. 362, no. 9381, August 2, 2003, p. 339.

237   "Oh. It's not hard at all. I go away from R&D": Maryann Gallivan, "A Perspective on Reengineering in Pharmaceutical Research and Development" speech to Financial Times Global Pharmaceutical Conference, October 20, 2003.

238   "Productivity is not something that this industry has been known for": John Symonds, "Keynote speech: Creating a Climate for Innovation," Ibid.
        "From about 1991 to 1996, we had a period of disequilibrium": Duncan Moore, "Strategic Dimensions of Risk Assessment," Ibid.
        "During that period, the default": Ibid.

5. *Independence for Generation Rx*

The question "What to do about pharma?" has become a growth industry in itself of late, with numerous conferences dedicated to

the topic scheduled for years to come. My focus on physician reform and regulatory reform was aided by Dr. Robert Goodman,
the founder of No Free Lunch, and by Larry Sasich, of Public Citizen. Ray Moynihan's work in the *British Medical Journal*, on the
subject of what he calls "physician entanglement," has also been
invaluable, as has the work of Massachusetts General Hospital's
David Blumenthal. On the subject of pharmacology, I have benefited from interviews with some of that field's leading lights,
among them Vanderbilt's Alastair Wood, the NIH's Art Atkinson, Indiana University's David Flockhart, and UCLA's Barbara
Levey. A conference held at UCLA in 2004 on the subject of phar-
macogenomics provided a wealth of ideas and sources as well,
some of which I summarize in this chapter. Ivan Illich consented
to two interviews, which I conducted in 1999, three years before
his death.

239   By the late 1990s, Goodman had grown convinced: Robert Good-
       man interview, November 15, 2004. See also Brendan I. Koerner,
       "Dr. No Free Lunch," *Mother Jones*, March/April 2003, p. 24, and
       David M. Studdert et al., "Financial Conflicts of Interest in Phy-
       sicians' Relationships with the Pharmaceutical Industry — Self-
       Regulation in the Shadow of Federal Prosecution," *New England
       Journal of Medicine*, vol. 351, no. 18, October 28, 2004, pp. 1891–
       1900.

240   "Our system would never tolerate judges taking money": Ray
       Moynihan, "Who Pays for the Pizza? Redefining the Relation-
       ships Between Doctors and Drug Companies. 2: Disentangle-
       ment," *British Medical Journal*, vol. 326, May 31, 2003, p. 1195.
       "model oath for the new physician . . . I will make medical deci-
       sions": Quoted in Ibid.

241   "That . . . presupposes that some of the most well-off": Quoted in
       Ibid.
       "Can you think of any other profession": William Vodra inter-
       view, March 20, 2003.

246   "therapeutic drug monitoring": Arthur Atkinson interview,
       March 3, 2004.
       "It ends up being [chaired by] someone who is very junior": Ibid.

247   "Does the drug work well enough to justify the bet?": Alastair
       Wood interview, July 24, 2002.

248   "yield a powerful set of molecular diagnostic methods": William
       E. Evans and Howard L. McLeod, "Pharmacogenomics — Drug
       Disposition, Drug Targets, and Side Effects," *New England Jour-
       nal of Medicine*, vol. 348, no. 6, February 6, 2003, pp. 538–49. See

also Yoseph Caraco, "Genes and the Response to Drugs," *New England Journal of Medicine*, vol. 351, no. 27, December 30, 2004, pp. 2867–69.

248   "It would be possible to genotype in trials": Alastair Wood interview, July 24, 2002.

249   "rational prescribing": David Flockhart interview, March 8, 2004. See also his Web site at www.medicine.iupui.edu/clinical/flockhart.htm.
     "One of the great traditional poisons": Ivan Illich interview, May 1999.

250   "Yes, we suffer pain, we become ill, we die": Jerry Brown, "Obituary for Ivan Illich," www.oaklandnet.com, December 2002.

254   "In work so taxing, moderation would be the best safeguard": Bernardino Ramazzini, *Diseases of Workers* (Birmingham, Ala.: Classics of Medicine Library, special edition, 1983). See also G. Franco, "Ramazzini and Workers' Health," *Lancet*, vol. 354, September 4, 1999, p. 858.

Index

Abbott Laboratories, 30, 36, 127

abbreviated new drug application (ANDA), 22

abuse of drugs. *See* drug abuse

Accupril, 100, 103, 104

Accutane, 212

ACE inhibitors, 58, 151, 194–96, 215. *See also* Prinivil

acetaminophen, 174. *See also* Tylenol

acid reflux. *See* gastroesophageal reflux disease

acne. *See* Accutane

ADD. *See* attention deficit disorder

addiction, 63, 90, 159–60

ADHD. *See* attention deficit hyperactivity disorder

adolescents. *See* youth

Advair, 124–25

adverse effects: and advertisements, 43, 48, 51, 52, 54; drug-drug interactions, 215, 216–18; gastrointestinal damage, 188, 189, 191, 197–201; heart damage, 3, 55, 163, 186–88, 189–91; liver damage (*see* drug-induced liver injury; liver: failure); lung or pulmonary damage, 187, 196–97; muscle tissue damage, 192, 194; need for surveillance systems, 243. *See also* addiction; death; suicide; *specific drugs and drug brand names*

advertisements: brief summary requirement, 43, 51, 52, 54; celebrities in, 54, 113, 188; creation of the drug distribution system, 31–55; FDA warning letters for deceptive, 55, 73, 93; first DTC campaign, 42–44; Latino-targeted, 109, 177, 180; in medical journals, 15, 32, 42, 60, 109; in newspapers and magazines, 112; by physicians, 12; reform, 243–44; state ban on, 12

African Americans, 195

aging, 5–6, 71, 73, 74, 215, 217. *See also* elderly

AIDS, 26, 27, 74

akathisia, 203, 204

albuterol, 69

alcohol, 101, 164, 185

allergies, 43, 160. *See also* Claritin; Flonase

Allnutt, Bob, 26, 29

alternative medicine, 14, 167

Alzheimer's disease, 162

AMA. *See* American Medical Association

Amaryl, 175, 177, 179

Ambien, 156, 158

American Association of Advertising Agencies (AAAA), 48–49, 52

American Association of Retired Persons (AARP), 226, 232

American Cancer Society, 26

American College of Gastroenterology, 72

American Diabetes Association, 26

American Home Products (AHP), 35, 51, 187–88

American Infertility Association, 119

Greg Critser is a longtime chronicler of the modern pharmaceutical industry and the politics of medicine. His columns and essays on the subject have appeared in the *New York Times, Harper's Magazine,* the *Wall Street Journal,* the *Los Angeles Times,* the London *Times,* and elsewhere. Critser is the best-selling author of *Fat Land: How Americans Became the Fattest People in the World,* which the American Diabetes Association called "the definitive journalistic account of the modern obesity epidemic."

ALSO BY GREG CRITSER

FAT LAND

*How Americans Became
the Fattest People in the World*

"Critser takes us seamlessly through the supersizing of
the American public . . . An in-depth, well-researched, and
thoughtful exploration of the fat boom in America."
— BOSTON GLOBE

In this disarmingly funny and truly alarming book, jour-
nalist Greg Critser investigates the many disparate factors
of American life — including class, politics, culture, economics, and the latest in medical research — that have con-
verged and conspired to place us among the fattest people
on the planet. *Fat Land* is "a medical wake-up call for the
nation . . . Incisive and compassionate" (Francine Kauf-
man, M.D., president, American Diabetes Association).

ISBN-13: 978-0-618-38060-2
ISBN-10: 0-618-38060-4

Visit our Web site:
www.marinerbooks.com.